The
ARCHETYPE
DIET

Reclaim Your Self-Worth and
Change the Shape of Your Body

DANA JAMES, MS, CNS, CDN

AVERY

an imprint of Penguin Random House

New York

AVERY

an imprint of Penguin Random House LLC
375 Hudson Street
New York, New York 10014

Copyright © 2018 by Dana James, MS, CNS, CDN
Foreword copyright © 2018 by Mark Hyman

Penguin supports copyright. Copyright fuels creativity, encourages diverse
voices, promotes free speech, and creates a vibrant culture. Thank you for buying an
authorized edition of this book and for complying with copyright laws by not reproducing,
scanning, or distributing any part of it in any form without permission. You are supporting
writers and allowing Penguin to continue to publish books for every reader.

Most Avery books are available at special quantity discounts for bulk purchase for sales promotions,
premiums, fund-raising, and educational needs. Special books or book excerpts also can be created
to fit specific needs. For details, write SpecialMarkets@penguinrandomhouse.com.

ISBN 9780735213760
Ebook ISBN 9780735213777

Printed in the United States of America

1   3   5   7   9   10   8   6   4   2

Book design by Gretchen Achilles

This is for every woman who has felt the pain of not enough—not pretty enough, not skinny enough, not important enough, and not different enough. You are not alone. May this book be a catalyst for deep self-discovery and complete self-acceptance.

CONTENTS

═══

PART III

THE SIX Rs TO HEAL YOUR MIND

The human body is one of the most complex systems on the planet, and not all bodies are the same. Anyone who has tried and struggled on a diet knows that what works for one person may not work for you; you have a unique body chemistry that needs to be addressed differently, and, without considering the hidden factors that may be affecting your ability to lose weight, you will continue to struggle. This is what functional medicine is all about: looking beyond the basics to determine what is right for each individual.

This, of course, presents an obvious problem with the vast majority of diets: by prescribing one set of specific recommendations for everyone, they fail to account for the multitude of factors that may be complicating one's ability to lose weight and rebalance her body. That is what makes Dana James's *The Archetype Diet* so revolutionary: by offering four diets designed for four different body types, she gives women the tools they need to first identify their bodies' specific needs and then follow a program that meets those needs completely.

I have known James for more than a decade, and this book beautifully captures the work she has been doing with her clients since she began her functional medicine practice. She has helped thousands of women reshape their bodies and reclaim their health, and now she offers a road map that anyone can use to do the same.

James also acknowledges that our diets affect more than just the shape of our bodies. Rooted in the principles of functional medicine, *The Archetype Diet* seeks to rebalance all of the systems that affect our health. Channeling the power of food as medicine, James understands that what we eat not only affects how much we weigh or what our body looks like but also how we feel and function overall. Diet plays a role in everything from digestion and immune response to skin conditions and hormone levels. Getting the balance right can be enormously tricky, but James cuts through the confusing, often conflicting advice that would-be dieters often encounter in favor of sound, pragmatic, and scientific facts about how food affects our health. Debunking the myths surrounding what makes a food "good" or "bad," she encourages women to let go of their fears around food in order to embrace the power real food has to heal our bodies.

James also goes beyond the physical to explore the very real body-mind connection so often overlooked by traditional diet plans. Although we are still only beginning to understand the connection between our diets and our minds, it's no secret that what we eat affects how we think and feel. Significant research has demonstrated how eating the right foods can increase our energy, boost the metabolism, combat depression and anxiety, and manage hormone levels, as well as a variety of other things that directly contribute to our overall mental state. As a functional medicine physician, I've dedicated my career to helping patients uncover this link within their own bodies so that they can radically improve their physical, mental, and emotional health.

But as James reveals in *The Archetype Diet*, the mind-body connection works in reverse as well. Just as how we eat affects how we think and feel, how we think and feel affects how we eat. While anyone who has ever struggled with a diet is familiar with the concept of emotional eating,

James shows how this cycle goes even deeper, beginning with some of our earliest memories and affecting our eating behaviors in ways we may not even notice.

Recognizing how our deepest, most ingrained thoughts and emotions influence our relationship with food, James developed her Archetype Model through her deep understanding that, just as women's bodies are different, so, too, are the reasons they eat the way they do. Without taking the time to explore the hidden motivations driving their eating behaviors, even the most motivated dieters will struggle. True, sustainable, lifelong health requires addressing the mind alongside the body and being compassionate with yourself as you seek to make meaningful change.

Ultimately, what makes *The Archetype Diet* so remarkable is not simply that it will help you lose weight (which it will). It's that it will help you attain a level of self-awareness and self-acceptance that will make it easier for you to not only stick to your diet, but to live the life you most truly want to live. Releasing yourself of the destructive emotions, habits, and behaviors will give you the freedom to move through the world with vitality in a body that supports your every move.

—**Mark Hyman, MD,**
director of the Cleveland
Clinic Center for Functional Medicine
and *New York Times* bestselling author

How Your Mind Shapes Your Body

═══

I know what I'm supposed to eat, but I just can't seem to lose weight."

This is the most common refrain I hear from my female clients. As a board-certified nutritionist and functional medicine practitioner with offices in Manhattan and Los Angeles, I have worked with more than three thousand women of all ages, sizes, and socioeconomic backgrounds. These clients come to me because, no matter what they do, they can't seem to change the shape of their bodies and are plagued by physical ailments from lack of energy to breakouts to perpetual bloating. They've tried every diet, detox, and exercise program under the sun, and while they might achieve some measure of success, they inevitably plateau or succumb to old habits that caused them to gain weight in the first place.

These are educated women who know that eating pizza and drinking soda won't help them lose weight, and they haven't touched these foods in years (okay, maybe a bite or sip or two after a few glasses of wine, but that's it!). At the same time, they're ashamed that their appearance matters so much to them. Shouldn't they, as empowered, twenty-first-century women, be focusing on their careers and their families instead of stressing over a bit of belly fat or the shape of their thighs?

This is where traditional diet plans fail most women. They focus exclusively on the physical—what and how much to eat—without acknowledging the role that your emotions play in helping you stick to a plan. Losing weight (and keeping it off) is only partly a physical process. Yes, what you eat (or don't eat) matters, but the main reason so many women struggle with food (despite knowing better) is psychological.

In the more than ten years that I've been working with women, I have found that the number one factor that determines whether a woman will succeed on her diet—and be able to sustain it over time—is where she sources her self-worth from. Whether she's a successful woman who rewards herself with a glass of wine (or three) every night after another long day at the office, or a kind and caring woman who finds herself in the kitchen at ten p.m. eating leftovers because she didn't have time to sit down and eat a real meal since everyone else's needs came before her own, these women have developed a dysfunctional relationship with food that prevents them from achieving their goals—dietary and otherwise. It may sound like a stretch—how is it possible that our feelings about ourselves can so profoundly affect what our body looks like or how much fat we put on—but time and again I've seen this pattern in my clients.

Here's what I mean. How you feel affects how you behave—including the way you eat—and the results eventually show on your body. You already know this intuitively. When you feel worthy of love and acceptance, you radiate confidence and energy and move through the world with ease. You take pleasure in caring for yourself and are more present and purposeful in the choices you make, dietary and otherwise. When your self-worth takes a nosedive because you think you are not pretty enough or smart enough or simply not good enough, you retreat into patterns that you hope will make you feel better but rarely do. You might skip meals, comfort eat, reward eat, or restrict food to compensate for these feelings—and then beat yourself up for not being more disciplined. Before long, you've given up on even the best-laid diet plan.

The way we source our self-worth is determined very early in our lives, typically in childhood, and is therefore so fully integrated into our identities that it can be difficult, if not impossible, to see how it drives our behavior. If you believe that your value as a person depends on some external factor—like good looks, intelligence, making others happy, or being unique—you will always be drawn to behave in ways that you think will increase that value and this will often influence how you approach food.

Through my work with clients, I have found that there are four primary ways that women derive their self-worth, which I have distilled into four essential archetypes. Archetypes, as defined by Carl Jung, are patterns of instinctual behavior. The first archetype is the Nurturer, who values herself on her ability to care for others. While this is a lovely and much-needed trait, if she is not conscious of her behaviors, she can end up prioritizing other people's needs and feelings to the point where she is depleted and exhausted. The second archetype is the Wonder Woman, who is a powerful female that derives her sense of self from what she has achieved in life. But, in her quest to not be a "nobody," she can become overwhelmed and emotionally disconnected from others. The third archetype is the sensual and playful Femme Fatale, who sources her self-worth from her physical body. This can make her incredibly alluring—but debilitatingly self-conscious. The fourth archetype is the Ethereal, who is dreamy and creative but highly sensitive to the world, making her feel discombobulated and anxious.

Each of the archetypes embody a particular set of personality traits—positive and negative. The problem occurs when the primary archetype starts to hijack your actions and thoughts to the exclusion of other things that make for a balanced life. The more dominant your archetype is (i.e., the more your sense of self-worth is wrapped up in one particular facet of your life), the more its negative attributes will show up in your behaviors as you seek to validate yourself by acting in a way that supports your self-worth.

In many cases, this behavior will affect your approach to food as well. For example, if you're a Wonder Woman and measure your value through your accomplishments, you may work through dinner in an effort to meet a deadline or check one more task off your to-do list. When your stomach starts rumbling at nine p.m., you'll order Thai takeout and then kick yourself ten minutes later for sabotaging your diet. The next day, when the pressure of work starts building yet again, you'll repeat the cycle; your sense of self-worth and the emotions associated with it have won out, yet again, over your rational mind. This is all part of a cycle that can't be short-circuited simply by counting calories or skipping dessert:

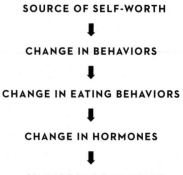

SOURCE OF SELF-WORTH

↓

CHANGE IN BEHAVIORS

↓

CHANGE IN EATING BEHAVIORS

↓

CHANGE IN HORMONES

↓

CHANGE IN BODY SHAPE

Traditional diet programs focus on how your eating behaviors affect your body—change your behavior, change your body shape—but they fail to consider the beginning of the behavior cycle. Yes, if you eat nutrient-dense foods that rebalance your hormones and help your body function properly, you will lose weight. But if you don't change how you *use* food (e.g., as a reward, distraction, desensitizer, comfort, or punishment), and more important, *why* you use food in this way, you will eventually revert to eating the same way you always have, ending up frustrated because you "know better." You can't master step three in the cycle until you understand how you got there. You need to start at step one—understanding where you source your self-worth from—if you want to have a balanced relationship with food and yourself.

Although every woman is unique, my work with my female clients has helped me identify certain patterns within each archetype. Specifically, women who source their self-worth from the same place tend to approach food in similar ways. In practical terms this means that, if they are out of balance and using food as a coping mechanism, they tend to suffer from the same physical imbalances and gain weight in the same way.

This discovery—the link between self-worth and body shape—made me realize that there's no such thing as a one-size-fits-all diet plan. Women need customized programs in order to address their distinct goals and challenges from both a physical and a psychological perspective. That is why I developed the Archetype Model, a road map of what to eat for weight loss, vitality, hormonal balance, and an overall sense of well-being. At its core, this model, which has become the foundation for how I treat all of my female clients, is about understanding *why* you eat the way you do (by identifying your archetype) and *how* that behavior affects your body. Then you adopt a food plan designed specifically for your archetype. The model also gives you the tools to examine how you came to source your self-worth in a particular way so you can free yourself from the hold that these beliefs had on you. The Archetype Model addresses the body and the mind, and it's all backed up by science and psychology.

While I designed the archetype meal plans specifically for women who want to lose weight, the ultimate goal of the Archetype Model is to dissolve the negative attributes associated with your archetype and integrate the best traits of *all* of the archetypes into your life. Every woman has the positive traits of all four archetypes within her, but because her dominant archetype can take over her life, she may not have expressed these positive traits in decades. A highly intellectual Wonder Woman, for example, may not value the intuition of the Ethereal, and therefore not nourish or cultivate her intuitive side. Nonetheless, intuition still exists within this Wonder Woman. As she decouples her sense of self-worth from her accomplishments, she will have the mind space to be able to nourish her intuition and any other traits that may have taken a backseat. It doesn't matter what your archetype is; when you cultivate your nurturing, playful, spiritual, and assertive side, you will become a more layered and balanced woman. You will stress less and life will flow with more grace and ease.

The Archetype Model draws on my knowledge of functional medicine, nutrition, and cognitive behavioral therapy to address the connections among our emotions, thoughts, behaviors, and physical body. But it is also inspired by my own experience struggling with weight loss. I grew up in one of Australia's prettiest beachside towns where all of the men and women were tanned, toned, and beautiful. While I was never clinically overweight, my body had curves and I didn't look like my leggy best friend, who was a swimwear model. Having come to believe that I would never be the prettiest, I decided that I would be smart instead. Over time, I began to view my achievements—academic and otherwise—as the barometer of my success and, consequently, my value as a woman. This behavior carried over into my adult life, and, even after studying nutrition for four years and knowing *exactly* what to eat, I unconsciously used food as a reward for working so hard. If you're a Wonder Woman, you will know this feeling all too well: the need to mindlessly eat something as you respond to the flood of emails. The food made me feel better about what I had to do; that is, keep working. It wasn't until I realized how my desire for success (a.k.a. my source of self-worth) was influencing my relationship with food that I was finally able to break this seemingly innocuous habit and achieve my desired weight and body shape.

This is exactly the type of breakthrough I want you to have as you read this book. In the chapters that follow, I will delve more deeply into each of the four archetypes to show how each one of them sources her self-worth and explain how the eating behaviors typical of each archetype show up on the body. I will help you identify your dominant archetype and provide practical tips for adjusting your diet to your body's particular needs, including a ten-day food plan, with recipes and nutritional supplements. I will debunk some of the most persistent myths surrounding food and explain how we *really* gain and lose weight in an effort to remove the fears and stigmas you may have developed in your efforts to balance your body. And I will guide you in examining your core childhood experiences so you can better understand the role they've played in your life. The goal is to transform your relationship with yourself and your body so you can achieve a healthier, happier relationship with food and become a more empowered and integrated woman.

Before we begin, I want to emphasize one important point. While I wrote this book for women who are struggling with their weight, the benefits of following the Archetype Model go well beyond weight loss. By becoming more fully aware of your innermost thoughts, beliefs, and fears and letting go of the behaviors that have altered your relationship with food, you will automatically have more energy to dedicate to more worthwhile pursuits. My clients have not only reshaped their bodies and found peace with food, they have also attained greater self-acceptance, reignited their self-worth, left depleting jobs to create successful businesses, and created more loving and deeply connected relationships.

What you can achieve when you eliminate the stress you've attached to food and your body is up to you to discover. My hope is that you will resolve the physical ailments you've struggled with (including your weight) and, in the process, uncover a more radiant, confident, energetic, and graceful version of you.

PART I

IDENTIFY

YOUR

ARCHETYPE

═══

CHAPTER 1

Which Archetype
Are You?

The meal plans and advice I provide in the rest of the book are designed to complement the archetype with which you identify the most. Before you can start to apply the principles of this book, you'll need to determine which archetype best encompasses the way you see yourself. You might assume you are a Wonder Woman by virtue of the demanding job you manage but at heart you are a Nurturer—you take on extra responsibilities because you don't want to disappoint anyone. You might assume you are a Femme Fatale because how you look is important to you, but you're actually an Ethereal who has taken on the mask of a Femme Fatale to fit in a society that overvalues physical appearance. Your archetype is not determined by what you *do*, it's *why* you do it. What is driving your behaviors? The answer lies in where you source your self-worth from.

The quiz below will help reveal the psychological underpinnings of your instinctive behavior and what motivates these behaviors. The questions are lighthearted, but it's important that you answer not as you'd *like* to respond but how you truly *would* respond in the situation presented. Select the one answer that best aligns with your likely response to the situation. Don't overthink it. If none of the options appeal to you, choose the most likely response. There is no right or wrong answer. No archetype is better than any other.

WHICH ARCHETYPE ARE YOU?

1. **PEOPLE DESCRIBE YOU AS:**

    a. Loving, giving, kind, and compassionate.

    b. Successful, smart, witty, and dynamic.

    c. Attractive, sexy, sparkly, and playful.

    d. Intuitive, sensitive, spiritual, and creative.

2. **ONE OF YOUR FAVORITE WAYS TO RELAX IS TO:**

    a. Bake cookies.

    b. Read a prizewinning book.

    c. Buy the latest color lipstick.

    d. Meditate to keep your mind calm.

3. **YOU FEEL YOUR BEST WHEN:**

    a. You care, love, or rescue others.

    b. You're recognized for your achievements.

    c. You're complemented on your looks, style, or taste.

    d. You're creatively expressing yourself.

4. **THE GREATEST SOURCE OF FRUSTRATION IN YOUR LIFE IS:**

    a. Your weight. It never seems to budge no matter what you do.

    b. Your love life. You can get so busy that meaningful romantic connections take a backseat to other priorities (even though you wish they didn't).

    c. Understanding of world events. You're so consumed by your own world that you can feel disconnected from political, social, and economic issues.

    d. Your finances. You have extraordinary visions but don't know how to make them profitable.

5.   **WHEN YOU GO OUT TO A NICE RESTAURANT, YOU ORDER:**

    a. Something a little carby, even though you know you shouldn't.

    b. Whatever you want. After a long, hard day you deserve it!

    c. Not much; there's no room for a poochy belly in *this* dress!

    d. A plate full of beans, rice, and tortilla wraps—as your friends look on in envy.

6.   **THE UNHEALTHIEST ASPECT OF YOUR RELATIONSHIP WITH FOOD IS:**

    a. You're a secret eater. You hide food from yourself only to "sneakily" eat it later in the day.

    b. You're generally good during the day, but you can blow it at night.

    c. You think about food and what it will do to your body 80 percent of the time.

    d. You frequently forget to eat.

7.   **YOU WORRY THAT YOUR PARTNER WILL:**

    a. Think you're needy.

    b. Be demanding and resent the time you spend working.

    c. Find someone more beautiful than you.

    d. Think you're weird.

8.   **THE LAST TIME YOU HAD A SERIOUS BREAKUP YOU:**

    a. Ate ice cream, then cried.

    b. Did everything possible to stay busy and didn't cry.

    c. Already had another suitor lined up.

    d. Cried then meditated until you made peace with the situation.

9. YOUR FAVORITE SCENT IS:

    a. Any fragrance with floral notes.

    b. A custom blend you import from France.

    c. Your man's pheromones.

    d. Palo santo.

10. AT THE COOL NEW APOTHECARY, YOU BUY:

    a. Heart tonic to strengthen your love.

    b. Brain tonic to enhance your mind.

    c. Sex tonic to intensify your lust.

    d. Intuition tonic to heighten your creativity.

11. WHEN SCANNING SOCIAL MEDIA YOU:

    a. Like everyone's posts.

    b. Feel a twinge of envy whenever someone posts about a new life milestone.

    c. Critique everyone's selfies.

    d. Post a photo from your most recent yoga retreat.

12. YOU TEND TO OVEREAT WHEN YOU'RE FEELING:

    a. Upset about something.

    b. Angry at someone, including yourself.

    c. Ugly and unattractive.

    d. Spacey and disconnected.

13. SOMETHING ABOUT YOU THAT YOU'D RATHER NOT ADMIT IS:

    a. Your health and finances have been compromised by putting others' needs before your own.

b. You feel guilty taking time off even though you know you need to relax.

c. You spend a lot of money on looking good.

d. You've struggled financially to pursue your creative passion.

14. IF YOU BREAK YOUR DIET, IT'S BECAUSE:

a. You don't want people to think you're a diva by ordering something different.

b. You've had a tough day and want to switch off with food or alcohol.

c. You're frustrated with yourself. You aren't losing fast enough.

d. You're feeling hypersensitive to the world and need carbs to dull the sensitivity.

15. WHEN YOU'RE UPSET, YOUR EATING STYLE IS TO:

a. Eat comfort food. Isn't that what everybody does?

b. Drink wine—that's your de-stress potion!

c. Control food—you either restrict or binge.

d. Ignore food. You don't care for food at the best of times.

16. AS A CHILD YOUR PARENTS MOST OFTEN PRAISED YOU FOR:

a. Helping around the house and looking after siblings.

b. Academic and athletic achievements.

c. Looking pretty.

d. Being different.

17. IF A FRIEND IS UNWELL, YOU:

a. Race over with chicken soup.

b. Stop by after work, answering emails on the way.

c. Bring her celebrity magazines and try to distract her by gossiping about your love lives.

d. Bring her a healing crystal and some herbal tea.

18. **YOU TEND TO CARRY BODY FAT:**

    a. Everywhere but especially on your upper thighs.

    b. Around your stomach.

    c. You don't have much—maybe five to ten pounds extra.

    d. You tend to be *too* skinny, but when you do gain weight, it's everywhere.

19. **IF A MAN YOU HAVE A CRUSH ON SENDS YOU A TEXT MESSAGE, YOU:**

    a. Respond right away, asking how his day was.

    b. Shoot back a witty response to keep the banter going.

    c. Respond with a flirtatious text.

    d. Wait until 11:11 p.m. to reply.

20. **WHEN INTERVIEWING FOR A JOB:**

    a. You send a thank-you note to everyone you spoke with.

    b. You say your greatest weakness is being a perfectionist (not that you really think it's a weakness).

    c. You dress impeccably.

    d. You would never take a job at a company with such a formal hiring process.

NOTE HOW MANY FOR EACH ANSWER HERE:

    a. _____
    b. _____
    c. _____
    d. _____

The highest score is your dominant archetype.

A: Nurturer   B: Wonder Woman   C: Femme Fatale   D: Ethereal

If you've identified your archetype correctly, you'll feel understood when you read the chapter about her that follows, like someone has read the inside of your mind—for better or for worse. You'll discover patterns you weren't consciously aware of. You'll also realize that you're not alone—there are plenty of other women with the same fears and the same motivators.

If your score on the quiz above is tied between two archetypes, read the chapters for each and see which archetype sits better with you. If you're still uncertain of your archetype, ask your friends. They'll know, just as you know theirs, your mother's, and your colleagues'. When your behavior is instinctive, you might not notice it, but other people do!

THE TRIANGLE OF BALANCE

While you will identify most strongly with one particular archetype, how strongly you identify with her will depend on whether you are in or out of balance. When you are fully in balance (a state I refer to as being at your "crown"), the characteristics of your primary archetype are integrated with positive attributes from the other archetypes. You are a complete woman. When you are out of balance, however, your archetype's characteristics—both positive and negative—are more prominent and will dictate your behaviors, from eating to relationships. When you are chronically out of balance, you'll behave in a way that bolsters your sense of self-worth to the detriment of other aspects of your life. You can do this by either amplifying your archetype's personality traits or withdrawing from them. The best way to visualize this is to think of an upright triangle. The highest point is the crown, while each point at the base represents amplification and withdrawal. For instance, a Femme Fatale might amplify her archetype by seeking validation and posting photos of herself in a bikini on social media. Or she might withdraw and be so afraid of showing off her body that the very thought of posting a selfie could have her running for the nearest Amish community. A Wonder Woman might work eighty hours a week and become the chief executive officer (CEO) of her company by amplifying her strength and ambition, or she could be spending eighty-hour weeks pushing paper for a superior because she's scared to go after a bigger job where she might be critiqued. She adapts by withdrawing from the positive traits of the archetype.

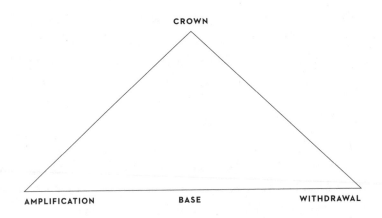

BODY TYPE, ARCHETYPE, AND DIET

Intuitively you know the diet that works for the supermodel isn't going to work for the supermom. These two women have different lives, different motivations, and, typically, different body shapes. Similarly, the diet that works for my binge-eating client is not going to work for my naturally lean yogini who often forgets to eat but has gained weight due to a metabolic issue. They need different sets of nutrients and therefore different meal plans to rebalance their unique physiologies.

The Archetype Model is a response to overly restrictive, one-size-fits-all plans that fail to consider how different bodies may respond to the same inputs in different ways. No other health issue is as complex as weight loss. It is a far cry from the "eat less, move more" philosophy that has permeated our culture for the past hundred years, nor is it as simple as eliminating one type of food in favor of others. Food, exercise, sleep, hormones, appetite, adrenals, thyroid, the gut microbiome, inflammation, genes, the environment, medication, habits, appetite, self-worth, subconscious thoughts, emotions, and stress can all affect how the body stores and burns fat. If you've ever wondered why you can't seem to lose weight even when you're exercising and eating right or why your best friend can eat heaping bowls of pasta without gaining a pound but your weight seems to ebb and flow as frequently as the tides, you're not crazy, or lazy, or undisciplined; the presiding weight loss equation of calories in/calories out is woefully inadequate.

What we call "fat" is actually adipose tissue that is composed of fat cells, inflammatory cells, toxins, and hormones. As hormones communicate with the adipose tissue about where to store fat, you can glean information about what is going on with your body biochemically by observing your body fat. This means, if you don't like your belly fat, thighs, or that overall layer of body fat, you can eat in a way that changes how hormones interact with the fat tissue so your body will stop storing fat in those places. Your personal trainer will tell you that you can't spot train, but you can eat in a way that does!

The Archetype Model is designed to address the different ways we store fat by recommending different food plans for each of the different archetypes. Since women who identify with a particular archetype source their self-worth from the same place, when they are out of balance they tend to share similar behaviors, including food behaviors, and, as a result, they tend to have the same hormonal imbalances that, in turn, cause them to gain weight in the same places.

For example, Nurturers often have higher levels of insulin and estrogen. Over time, too much insulin will slow her body's ability to burn fat so she'll end up carrying weight all over her body. Excess insulin can also trigger the production of estrogen, which directs fat to be stored on the upper thighs. Because of this, out-of-balance Nurturers tend to have a full, curvy body shape. Meanwhile, the successful Wonder Women, who fears being invalidated, dismissed, or perceived as irrelevant, tends to complain of excess belly fat, a sign that her body is producing too much cortisol, a hormone that spikes during times of stress. If left unregulated, this can lead to fatigue, adrenal depletion, and a thyroid imbalance—all of which can affect one's ability to lose weight. Out-of-balance Femme Fatales are petrified of gaining weight because they source their self-worth from their looks. Their weight often yo-yos back and forth depending on whether they are restricting food to lose weight or overeating out of shame or frustration. They may have too much cortisol, insulin, and/or estrogen and therefore take on a certain body shape depending on what they're eating. Ethereals are naturally thin and therefore don't gain weight as easily as the other archetypes, but if they feel depressed, anxious, or highly sensitive to the world around them, they can compensate by eating too many refined carbs. This wreaks havoc on their metabolism, causing them to appear "skinny fat"—not overweight but carrying a thin layer of pinchable fat over their thin muscles.

As the meal plans in this book are designed specifically to help women lose weight and lose fat from the areas that bother them the most, I've provided strict guidelines on portion size and serving frequency for each archetype. For instance, a Nurturer will benefit from limiting her intake of carbohydrates to decrease her insulin levels, thereby shrinking fat cells from all over her body. On the other hand, the naturally thin Ethereal can eat more unrefined carbohydrates than any of the other archetypes because these carbs help to free up more estrogen, which Ethereals tend to have too little of. A Wonder Woman with excess cortisol should avoid common food sensitivities, like gluten and dairy, since these act as physical stressors on the body and add to her already high stress load.

As you adjust to the new eating behaviors you will naturally adopt as you follow your archetype's meal plan and change your relationship with food, you may find that you can eat more without gaining weight. The goal here is not just to get you to a particular dress size, it's also to reexamine your approach to food so you come to see it as a source of nourishment instead of a source of fear, reward, comfort, or distraction.

One other side note: if you continue to have problems losing weight or find yourself suffering from some other physical ailment, consult with a functional medicine practitioner who can run tests to see what else might be going on in your body. While the archetype-specific meal plans are designed to take into consideration all parts of the body that can affect weight gain—thyroid, adrenals, gut microbiome, inflammation, hormones, and so on—you might have a specific condition that requires a more customized treatment. I trust that this book will help you no matter your physiology, but sometimes a one-to-one consultation is needed to make some small, subtle adjustments. Don't be afraid to ask for help.

Now that you've identified your dominant archetype, it's time to learn more about the personality traits and behavioral patterns associated with her so you can better understand how your sense of self-worth is influencing your behaviors. You'll discover how these thoughts and patterns affect your body shape as well as what foods you can eat to rebalance your hormones and decrease body fat.

Beyond that, when you read the other archetype chapters, you'll also come away with a greater understanding of the women in your life. When you know your mother's and daughter's archetypes, you'll know how best to respond to them because you're aware of what motivates them and what makes them vulnerable. Personalities clash and we get annoyed with people, particularly those close to us; but by understanding them, we won't take it personally and thus won't get so upset by the situation. By offering kindness instead of judgment, you create more cohesion and solidarity among women and strengthen the power of all women.

CHAPTER 2

The Nurturer

_____

Paige is vivacious, warm, and caring. She loves to be there for everyone—
and she is! She's an event planner who gives her all to her clients—even
the difficult, demanding ones whom she never seems able to please. She
wants everyone to be happy, but her constant people-pleasing is taking its
toll. She feels exhausted, bloated, and constipated. She's also carrying an
extra thirty pounds of body fat and can't seem to get rid of it no matter
how healthy she eats. (Though, if she's honest, she's been mindlessly eating sweets to comfort herself.) Her friends tell her to take time for herself,
but how is she supposed to say no to someone who needs something from
her? Paige is the quintessential Nurturer.

THE NURTURER AT HER CROWN:
EMPATHETIC AND DEPENDABLE

The Nurturer derives her sense of power from her ability to care for others.
She is known for her dependability, loyalty, and thoughtfulness and will drop

whatever she is doing to be there for family and friends. She'll take a three a.m. phone call from a bereft girlfriend because she wants to be there for her. She'll bake her partner's favorite lemon and olive oil cake just because. She'll surprise you with little gifts simply because they "made her think of you." Nurturers instinctively know what makes people happy, and they have a unique ability to make those around them feel special and supported.

Nurturers are empathetic and kind in a way that would be draining for any other archetype. A Nurturer doesn't need a reason to be generous; it's in her DNA—and her upbringing. The Nurturer is not a pushover, however. She's fiercely loyal, and if you upset those close to her, she will unfailingly protect them and you will feel her fury! The Nurturer is like the mother hen protecting her chicks, swooping in to guard her loved ones from harm.

When Nurturers are at their crown, they inspire others to be more loving, peaceful, and generous. We want Nurturers to be our mother figures—or mothers. We want them to hold us, care for us, and protect us. We want to nestle into the safety of their embrace and be warmed by their unconditional love and acceptance. Nurturers are nourishment. Nurturers are comforting.

Notable Nurturers include Oprah, Christina Hendricks, Adele, Jessica Alba, Amma "the hugging saint," Mother Teresa, Melanie Hamilton from *Gone With the Wind*, and your best friend, who is always there for you no matter what is going on in her life.

THE BELIEF SYSTEM: "I AM WORTHY BECAUSE OF HOW I CARE FOR YOU"

Caring for others is how the Nurturer sources her self-worth. She will often choose to become a healer, social worker, nurse, teacher, or personal assistant, as these careers offer the most opportunity to care for people.

Not disappointing others is so fundamental for the Nurturer that she can feel sick to her stomach if she thinks she has upset someone. She can ruminate and ruminate.

This belief system can show up in very subtle ways. My client Alicia found herself bewildered one day after ordering a bagel at a deli instead of the omelet she'd planned on. When she told me the ordering line was long, I knew what had happened; the omelet would take longer to make than the bagel, and she couldn't stand the thought of holding others up—even strangers—so she unconsciously sabotaged her diet without even realizing why. Her Nurturer had hijacked her conscious mind.

As much as the Nurturer prides herself on giving, she can find it extremely challenging to receive help, compliments, or just about anything that suggests she is herself in need of nurturing. I suspected my friend Natalie was a Nurturer. When we were away at a yoga retreat together, which she helped organize, I asked her if she had booked herself a massage. "Oh no," she said. "I want to make sure that everyone who wants a massage has one first, and then if there's still space, I'll take that spot." Natalie wasn't being grand or selfless but rather displaying the Nurturer's core belief: "You before me. I'm happy when you're happy." But Nurturers, like all of us, need to be cared for, too.

While being a parent necessitates nurturing, the state of motherhood doesn't define a woman as a Nurturer. To be the Nurturer, she must value her entire being on how she cares for people. If taking time out for herself feels self-indulgent, then she's likely a Nurturer, and an out-of-balance one at that.

CHILDHOOD PATTERNS:
NEGLECTED OR CODEPENDENT

A Nurturer may have been raised by a nurturing mother who instilled these feminine qualities in her daughter. If this was done in a healthy, non-codependent way, the young girl will have grown up to be a Nurturer whose crown is placed firmly on her head. This woman likes to see people happy and it makes her feel good to know she had a hand in that happiness. Her nurturing nature comes from a place of love rather than a sense of guilt or a need to be accepted by others.

All too often, however, the Nurturer was raised in an environment where her own mother's nourishment was absent due to work, a sick family member, a troubled marriage, an illness, drug use, alcoholism, or simply a lack of warmth. Because she was deprived of the maternal attention young girls need, she learned to fill this void by protecting and nurturing others, essentially taking on the role of the mother she lacked. Although the recipients of her nurturing could not make up for the failings of her own mother, she depended on them to give her the acceptance she so craved. By showing love to others, she hoped to get it in return.

Alexandria grew up with an alcoholic father and distraught mother who unintentionally deprived her daughter of love and affection. Alexandria responded by tending to her mother's needs and protecting her from her father's angry outbursts. Alexandria came to view her mother's attention as the reward she got for caring for and protecting her. Her self-worth became tied to pleasing others. Alexandria became a Nurturer.

Kerry's story is similar. She grew up in a single-parent household with two younger siblings. Her mother worked as a substitute teacher so she could support the children but was emotionally distant and felt uncomfortable expressing affection. Kerry wanted motherly love and thus felt betrayed. She sought solace in nurturing her siblings, which created a subconscious imprint that nurturing equals worthiness. Kerry, too, became a Nurturer.

If the Nurturer becomes a mother, she may overcompensate for the lack of maternal affection she experienced as a child by putting her children's needs before her own to the point of burnout. Or she might inadvertently develop codependent relationships with them, smothering them to the point that they feel pressured and constricted. This can cause her children to retreat from the Nurturer in order to escape the cloying affection and guilt cycle she has unintentionally created. In her misguided efforts to earn affection, the Nurturer may end up alienating those closest to her.

OUT OF BALANCE: "I DON'T WANT TO BE A BURDEN"

While a Nurturer derives pleasure and intimacy from giving attention to others, her positive traits of compassion and giving can become perverted when they are used as a tool for attention and self-worth. As with all archetypes, the coping strategy is either an amplification of or a withdrawal from these traits, and she can swing between these two extremes depending on the situation.

In the amplification, an out-of-balance Nurturer puts everyone else's needs before her own. She can give and give to others until she's depleted and broken. Saying "no" can feel like a betrayal of who she is, and she would rather exhaust herself than give someone a reason to think she was selfish. She can't prioritize where to spend her time, energy, and care, and the slightest flicker of upset in someone's eye will send her into healer mode. Her unconditional generosity becomes a kind of armor; "If I give and give, you'll see how loving I am and it will be impossible for you to reject me." This is not a conscious thought but one lodged deep in the Nurturer's psyche.

In the withdrawal, the Nurturer learns to hide. "If I just stay out of the way and don't make my presence felt, I won't be noticed, and I won't be a burden." These thoughts permeated her childhood and still show up today. The care the Nurturer desired as a child is still missing from her life. Where is the love for her? Where is the tenderness that she needs? Where is her nourishment? The Nurturer has deflected it and unconsciously set up patterns to make sure she is needed and missed when she's not around.

THE NURTURER ARCHETYPE: FIRST CHAKRA

The first chakra (root chakra) connects us to the earth. It makes us feel that we're part of the tribe. The first chakra is located near the rectum and is associated with the elimination of waste, negative thinking, and feeling isolated. It represents survival and physical and emotional security. When the Nurturer creates codependent relationships or stays in them for the sake of not disrupting the status quo, she's operating out of a destabilized first chakra. Her safety and survival are at stake. We can all feel a first chakra imbalance, but the Nurturer feels it more keenly.

Red is the color of the first chakra, so as a Nurturer you can use this color spectrum to rebalance yourself. Eat vibrant red foods such as organic watermelon, tomatoes, red bell peppers, guava, rhubarb, and beets to help free yourself from negative and self-doubting thoughts. Wear a bright red lipstick or paint your toenails lobster red when you want to feel more connected. Wear a red dress on a date to assert yourself. (There's a reason why red stilettos are associated with power: they connect the wearer to the first chakra and help stake your claim!) You can also wear red jewels to give yourself the strength to say no yet still feel part of the tribe.

EATING BEHAVIOR: "I'M AFRAID TO BE EMPTY"

Because the Nurturer can de-prioritize her own needs for the sake of others', she can neglect herself—including her health. She can feel that she doesn't have the time to cook herself a nutritious meal, particularly if it means a different meal from the rest of the family, let alone exercise, meditate, or get a proper night's sleep. The longer this goes on, the more she disconnects from her body. She learns to ignore her own hunger and physical symptoms. She gains weight but is too overwhelmed with the needs of her family, friends, and work colleagues to be concerned enough to change her eating. An out-of-balance Nurturer may only notice there's a problem after she experiences a health scare—being diagnosed with an autoimmune disease, a prediabetic warning from her physician, or seeing the scale hit the two-hundred-pound mark. However, unless she addresses how she values herself, any change she makes will be short-lived as she reverts to her protective patterns of being needed.

Since feeding others is a universal form of caring, it's not surprising that food becomes the Nurturer's solace when she needs to be comforted. If she hasn't taken the time to understand the motivations behind her behaviors, she can feel empty and unconsciously seek to fill the void left by the absence of unconditional love she perceived in her childhood, through food. More than any other archetype, how a Nurturer eats is reflective of her emotional state. She will comfort-eat, binge-eat, get caught in addictive food patterns, and struggle in social situations. At shared meals, she can pile her plate high, fearful that she may not get enough. She'll prepare dinner for her children or partner but forget about herself. When she's left to her own devices, she'll eat cereal, yogurt, or whatever her children left behind on their dinner plates rather than devote time to cooking for herself.

A Nurturer may also be a secret eater. Sometimes it's so secret, she won't even admit it to herself. My client Angie would buy cookies "for the kids" and hide them on the top shelf of the kitchen cabinet so she couldn't see them or reach them without a stool. One day her daughter discovered her standing on the stool eating cookies and said, "Mommy, if you don't want to eat them, why don't you store them even higher so you really can't reach them?" The innocence of her daughter's observation snapped Angie out of her bizarre (but not uncommon) behavior.

A Nurturer can struggle with a diet. When her comfort foods are removed, her emotions will surface and, if she doesn't have skills to process those emotions, she can feel overwhelmed and go back to eating because it calms her. The Nurturer is the archetype most likely to complain that she feels addicted to certain foods. However, it's more likely that she's addicted to the act of eating. Eating is her pacifier.

If you are a Nurturer, you must be willing to recognize the emotions you're trying to hide in order to find success on a diet. You need to learn to sit with the discomfort of these feelings and not use food to console yourself. It's not the food, per se, that's the issue; it's the unwillingness to examine the uncomfortable emotions. Once you no longer use food to block the emotion, you'll gain insight into why you've been viscerally pulled toward certain foods.

My client Beverly ran a swimming pool company and felt financially responsible for the forty employees, most of whom were family. She didn't trust anyone to assist her and worked until ten p.m. most nights and weekends, although she resented the long hours. Hard as she tried to swallow the anger, her physical body let it show. When we first met, Beverly weighed four hundred pounds. When I asked her to remove certain foods from her house, she did so reluctantly. One morning she discovered a trail of bread crumbs leading from her kitchen out to her car, and although she had no recollection of doing so, she realized that sometime during the night she'd eaten a dozen rolls meant for an office party that she'd left in the backseat.

Simply telling Beverly what not to eat was not enough to help her lose weight. She needed to come to terms with the frustration and resentment she was feeling and trust that asking for help wasn't a burden on someone else. She needed to learn how to honestly express herself. If you are a Nurturer who has been programmed to believe, "I need to take care of everyone," this can be a profound shift in your thinking.

THE CHALLENGE FOR NURTURER: IT'S SAFE TO SAY NO

As the Nurturer fears offending people, saying no doesn't always feel safe. Since she may have grown up in a household with absent or troubled parents, saying yes to chores—doing the laundry, making dinner, watching siblings—was how she earned attention. She believes, erroneously, that if she doesn't do something, it won't get done. As there were rarely people she could rely upon as a child, she doesn't trust others to be there for her today. This belief has become so ingrained into her subconscious that she still says yes to almost any favor or task asked of her.

This imprint is not just psychological, it's also physical. Her brain has been wired to care for others. An unpredictable childhood has sensitized her to other people's moods. A slight change in someone's tone of voice can put her on high alert, and she instinctually jumps in to solve the problem.

In order to ascend to your crown, you must believe with every single cell in your body—not just your rational mind—that it's okay (and safe) to say no and that, just because someone else has a problem, doesn't mean you need to solve it. Similarly, things will get done, even if you don't make it happen personally. The belief that it won't get done if you don't do it is a residue from childhood. Ask for help and you'll be surprised by the support you receive. Start by learning to say yes whenever someone offers you help. Accepting assistance—whether it's from a spouse, a friend, a co-worker, or anyone else in a position to give it—is not a sign that you are a burden but an acknowledgment that you deserve to be nurtured, too. Be patient with the process as you get used to it, and trust that people are genuinely offering to help you without conditions. As you learn to receive help from others, you will start to feel safe with others giving to you and will learn to be okay with not doing it all by yourself.

To be clear, accepting help does not mean you need to stop giving.

Showing affection for others and caring for them is your gift and it should be celebrated. But choose the recipients wisely. Pause before you bestow your kindness, time, love, or money. Ask yourself if this person genuinely needs your help or if they can handle things on their own. The more you consider this question, the easier it will become to respond accordingly without feeling guilty. This is where understanding the other archetypes is helpful. Wonder Women and Femme Fatales are the most resilient and resourceful and are more likely to ask if they need help; you don't need to offer it to them. Take this time and give it to yourself. Ethereals tend to be more reserved and may not ask for your help. Check in with them and ask if they require assistance before you jump in. It's not your responsibility to rescue them.

As you ascend to your crown, you will learn to love deeply without sacrificing yourself. You will become lighter (physically and emotionally) by not carrying the responsibilities of others. Every cell in your body will know that you are loved for who you are, not because of what you give to or do for others. Embracing the positive attributes of the other archetypes will help you achieve balance and rise to the crown.

- Channel your inner Femme Fatale by caring for your physical body. Buy that bright red Tom Ford lipstick not only because you look hot wearing it but because the color helps to rebalance your emotional state. Remember, caring for others does not mean neglecting yourself.
- Tap into your inner Ethereal to learn how to listen to your intuition and discern who and what will bring joy to your life.
- Let Wonder Woman imbue you with the strength to say no so you have more time to dedicate to yourself.

When you layer in these attributes, you will transform from a Nurturer seeking to heal your childhood wounds to a woman who heals the world with her loving presence, compassion, dignity, and nobility.

THE NURTURER'S FOOD PRESCRIPTION

Understanding the Nurturer's biochemistry—how your body functions and how your environment and diet affect those functions—will help you realize that your struggle to lose weight is not a reflection on you as a person but rather a sign of hormonal imbalances that interfere with weight loss. Like all of the archetypes, where you store body fat gives clues as to the hormones at play. Nurturers tend to store fat all over their bodies, and you may feel like you are wearing a fat suit, which you wish you could just step out of. Over time, if you don't pay attention to your physical body, you'll start to store fat on your upper thighs and upper arms. The more out of balance you are, the more body fat you store. The good news is, subtle changes to your diet will have a profound impact on speeding up weight loss and directly targeting fat loss from your problem areas.

Before we explore your unique biochemistry, I want to emphasize that the goal for a Nurturer should not be to become ultra-thin. A Nurturer is never going to look like an Ethereal, and if you attempt that, you will set yourself up for years of disappointment. I want you to embrace your strong, womanly body. It is extremely feminine and sensual and projects a sense of trust. And take some solace in the fact that many the Ethereal wishes she had a Nurturer's boobs and butt!

HORMONAL IMBALANCES—INSULIN AND ESTROGEN

The Nurturer's dominant hormones are insulin and estrogen. If you've read any diet book over the past twenty years (and I know you've read many!), you'll know that the hormone insulin tells the body to store *excess* carbs as body fat. Exactly what comprises "excess" carbs will depend on your level of exercise and how efficient your body is at regulating your glucose levels. Most out-of-balance Nurturers are not good at regulating their glucose levels and often have insulin resistance. Because your body preferentially stores glucose as body fat, you tend to have a curvy and full body shape.

When you grab a muffin on the way to work because you didn't have time to make breakfast, your body will store those carbs as fat and it will not burn body fat for several hours. This muffin will mess with your sugar levels, and you will end up—in a cruel biochemical irony—feeling hungrier because your muscle cells are starved for glucose. However, if you ate an omelet for breakfast (even if it had the same number of calories as the muffin), you'd burn fat instead of storing it because the protein would stimulate the production of glucagon, one of the body's fat-burning hormones that also helps to suppress the appetite. This is why counting calories as your only dietary guideline is ineffective. You must also consider where those calories are coming from and which hormones are being triggered.

The Nurturer also tends to have higher levels of estrogen. You may be genetically programmed to produce more estrogen or may not be metabolizing estrogen well, thereby causing more active forms of estrogen to stay in your body for longer. Excess insulin also increases the amount of freely available estrogen in the body. The higher the level of free estrogen, the more it can communicate with fat cells. Researchers have found that there are different estrogen receptors in the glutes versus the abdominal area, which can partially explain why there's a different distribution of fat on different women.[1] If you are experiencing elevated levels of estrogen, then you will start to store fat on your hips and upper thighs, which have more estrogen receptors than other parts of the body.[2]

The excess estrogen increases the risk of fibroids, endometriosis, and breast cancer since the tissue in these areas is stimulated by estrogen. It also contributes to premenstrual syndrome (PMS), polycystic ovary syndrome (PCOS), and unmanageable perimenopausal symptoms, and it can suppress the thyroid function, making it even more difficult for you to lose weight. I observe more severe thyroid imbalances in Nurturers than in Wonder Women because many Nurturers have learned to comfort-eat. These comfort foods increase insulin, interfere with estrogen levels, and suppress active thyroid hormones, making the whole damn situation much worse! The Nurturer's signaling system is out of whack, and until she repairs it, she will continue to gain weight, feel fatigued, be hungry, and experience symptoms of estrogen dominance.

AUTOIMMUNE DISEASES

Autoimmune diseases such as Hashimoto's and fibromyalgia are also more likely in the Nurturer than other archetypes. This is partially due to her pull toward more carbohydrate-based foods when she is upset but also due to unexpressed emotions and negative childhood events such as an alcoholic parent, a sick family member, or physical or emotional abuse. According to the Adverse Childhood Experiences (ACE) study, one of the largest studies on childhood trauma and adult outcomes ever undertaken, just one of these events increases the chance of being hospitalized for an autoimmune disease by 20 percent.[3] If you have two or more ACEs, your risk increases by 70 percent. While I don't cover specific autoimmune diseases in depth in this book, the tools you'll find in these pages can help to reduce their severity.

THE FEARS

As a Nurturer you may find that weight loss is slow, not because you don't want to lose weight but because you resist change. You are genuinely scared to be hungry and fearful of making changes that might cause this. If the Nurturer doesn't feel safe with her eating plan, she can find herself secretly eating and end up stuck in a guilt-shame cycle. But this isn't all in your mind; you *will* be hungrier than the other archetypes, which is why it's vital that you follow the meal plan I've created for your archetype since it has been specifically designed to reduce hunger.

You must also learn to trust yourself not to fall into an overeating spiral at the first hint of temptation or hunger. You are not weak or broken or undisciplined. Your desire to please and care for others has, over time, led you to form habits and behavioral patterns that allow you to put others' needs before your own. This is why it's essential for you—and all of the archetypes—to examine your childhood wounds and how you source your self-worth in an effort to identify the root causes of your eating (and other) behaviors and take the steps to change them. Since your mind is your biggest barrier—often telling you that you have no time for yourself—you'll need to work diligently through Part III about healing the mind so you can silence these false voices. Taking care of yourself is not a selfish act but rather a way for you to become more physically and emotionally resilient. When you feel restored, you can give more freely to others because your love comes from a place of abundance, not depletion. You are able to receive from others as much as you give to others. You become whole.

THE NURTURER'S MEAL PLAN

Since your biochemistry makes you the most sensitive of all of the archetypes to carbs, your diet is slightly more limited than those of the other archetypes. Remember, though, it is designed to help you lose weight, rebalance your hormones, and repair your metabolism. You should immediately feel more energized and see a reduction of inflammation in your body. Eating this way consistently will also give you the vitality and body shape you've desired for so long without you having to follow a complicated or overly restrictive diet ever again.

The guidelines below outline the general principles around which you should structure your meals. A ten-day plan, which incorporates these concepts, is in Chapter 13.

Step 1: Improve Your Daily Eating Regimen

1. Start each morning with an elixir to boost your metabolism. In spring and summer, drink the juice of an entire lemon in 12 ounces of cool water. In fall and winter, drink a warming ginger tea.
2. Eat a protein-based breakfast; no oats, cereal, toast, or muffins.
3. Be sure lunch and dinner each consist of six ingredients: three vegetables, one protein, and two fats. Do not include carbs like sweet potatoes, beans, rice, or quinoa. These meals should look like the food plate on page 31.
4. Don't skip meals or snacks, even if you are busy. They are essential for stabilizing your blood-sugar levels and decreasing hunger.
5. Wind down your evenings with a tea specifically designed for your biochemistry (included below).
6. Supplement as recommended below to reset your metabolism and rebalance your hormone levels.

Step 2: Choose the Right Foods

Specific foods can help to rebalance the Nurturer's physical and emotional state. These suggestions should be followed in conjunction with the general recommendations made in Part II to address your particular hormonal concerns.

1. Eat at least one cruciferous vegetable daily. These include kale, arugula, watercress, broccoli, Brussels sprouts, cabbage, cauliflower, collard greens, Swiss chard, and bok choy. Cruciferous vegetables help to detoxify estrogen and decrease insulin resistance. Add

broccoli to a stir-fry, make a cauliflower soup for lunch, or try grilled fish with a summer slaw made with purple and green cabbage.

2. Eat one red fruit or vegetable daily. Since red is associated with the Nurturer's root chakra, incorporating red fruits and vegetables into your diet will support your emotional stability.

3. Skip carbs except at your pleasure meal. Since you are prone to insulin resistance, you need to limit your carbohydrate intake. The carbs in your diet should come principally from vegetables. This means vegetable soup instead of lentil soup, raw zucchini noodles instead of pasta, and cauliflower rice instead of grain bowls. Nurturers can eat up to two 1-cup servings of fruit per day (except bananas, which are too sugary for the Nurturer).

4. Eat 5 ounces of clean animal protein at both lunch and dinner. This portion size is slightly larger than what I recommend for the other archetypes because the additional protein will help decrease your hormone-induced hunger.

5. Eat lighter forms of protein. Lean toward a pescatarian diet, with fish, eggs, hemp seeds, and plant-based protein powders as your preferred protein sources. These are easier to digest and are energetically lighter, making you feel less stagnant and inflamed. Eat organic poultry when these protein sources are unavailable.

6. Eat red meat no more than twice per month. Red meat, such as beef, lamb, pork, and game, is the most grounding type of protein, and since most Nurturers already feel grounded and want to feel lighter, it's best to eat red meat sparingly.

7. Avoid tofu and tempeh. Because soy has a weak estrogenic effect, Nurturers should avoid eating tofu and tempeh. Small amounts of miso and tamari (wheat-free soy sauce) are fine since they are used for flavor and not as a protein source.

8. Avoid nuts and nut butters. Most of your fat should come from seeds, olives, avocados, and olive oil. Nuts are too energetically

dense for the Nurturer and can make you feel stuck and stagnant. The exception is Brazil nuts, which contain nutrients that support a healthy thyroid function. You can eat four Brazil nuts as a snack.

9. Use spices. Spices like cardamom, cinnamon, ginger, and turmeric help fire up the metabolism. Add turmeric to your eggs at breakfast or a dash of cinnamon to your morning coffee.

10. Avoid dairy. Dairy has the propensity to stimulate insulin, making it more difficult for you to lose weight. This includes yogurt, feta cheese, whey protein powder, and all other foods and beverages made from cow, sheep, or goat's milk. The only exception is your treat meal, which is discussed in Chapter 12.

Foods that rebalance the Nurturer: grilled fish, raw salads, seeds, cruciferous vegetables, and warming spices as well as red fruits and vegetables.

Foods that should be kept to a minimum: grains, legumes, root vegetables, nuts, red meat, dairy, and sweets.

THE NURTURER'S TEA

This tea was developed specifically for the Nurturer by the Ayurvedic practitioner Nadya Andreeva. It contains hibiscus, which helps decrease cellular inflammation and suppresses the appetite. The cardamom reduces swelling while the cloves and ginger are stimulating to help fire up your metabolism. Drink a cup in the evening to help you release the tension of the day. This recipe will make one 12-ounce cup of tea, but you can mix the ingredients in bulk and store them in an airtight container.

2 tablespoons dried hibiscus flowers

1-inch piece of fresh ginger, thinly sliced

5 green cardamom pods

1 whole clove

Combine the ingredients in a small pot with 12 ounces of hot water. Steep for 5 minutes, then strain into a tea cup. Add more hot water if the tea is too strong.

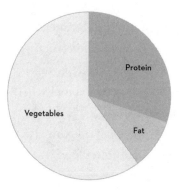

THE NURTURER'S FOOD PLATE

Step 3: Supplement Strategically

I have found the following supplements to be the most helpful in bringing my Nurturers back into balance. I have provided recommendations on where to find these in Appendix C, "Resources."

- **A glucose-regulating supplement:** Choose one that contains green tea, vanadium, black pepper, cinnamon, chromium, alpha lipoic acid, magnesium, and gymnema sylvestre. These nutrients improve glucose levels and can help reset the insulin response.[4] Take daily.

- **EPA/DHA (Omega-3):** Omega-3s have consistently been shown to improve blood-sugar regulation and insulin sensitivity.[5] It's believed that they increase adiponectin (a protein that regulates glucose), reduce inflammation in the fat cells, and improve how the receptor cells listen to the metabolic hormones. Take 1,000 mg of the active form of omega-3s EPA and DHA daily.

- **L-carnitine:** This is an amino acid that helps shuttle fat into the mitochondria to be burned as fuel.[6] It helps switch you from a carbohydrate burner to a fat burner.[7] This means you'll preferentially burn body fat (not glycogen) during your workout and you'll be less hungry after you exercise. Take 3 grams in a powder form so that it can easily be mixed into water and consumed.

- **DIM:** DIM is the key component in cruciferous vegetables that helps to metabolize estrogen to a weaker form.[8] Take 300 mg daily.

- **B complex:** Take an activated B complex to help boost energy levels and regulate hormone levels. Look for the activated forms, which include L-5-MTHF (folate), pyridoxine HCl (B6), and methylcobalamin (B12). Take one daily after food.

As you ascend to your crown and rebalance your physical body, you can relax these meal guidelines and add some starchy carbs back into your diet, starting with ½ cup at lunch and at dinner. You can also reintroduce red meat up to once a week, and nuts according to the portion sizes suggested on page 31. If you find your weight stagnating, return to the baseline program outlined above until you are back on track, then reintroduce these foods more gradually.

EXERCISE SOLUTIONS FOR THE NURTURER

Because the Nurturer often feels heavy and inflamed, an exercise program that boosts her metabolism is best for her. Ideal types of exercise include the rebounder, running, boxing, HIIT (high-intensity interval training), circuit training, and dance. Do any combination of these four days a week and take a yoga class once a week. This is not to say that slower movement classes, like a barre class, won't work for you (it's certainly better than nothing), but it's less effective than the high-intensity classes. If you love barre class or Pilates, go up to three times a week, but you must add three other types of exercise the rest of the week. The goal of exercise for a Nurturer is to increase fat burning, boost the metabolism, boost the thyroid function, and circulate the lymphatic fluid.

CHAPTER 3

The Wonder Woman

I was sixteen years old and a gun was pointed at my head. This was not some teenage suicide game; there was an armed robbery in progress at the produce store where I worked (yes, even then I liked vegetables). I grew up in a beautiful, safe, beachside town in Australia, so I was not prepared for such violence. People here carried surf boards, not guns!

Once my initial shock subsided, I started to fill the beige bank bag with money as the man in the hood had demanded. When he tried to grab it out of my hand, I snarled at him and spat, "I'm not finished yet!" continuing to fill the bag with money. Only a Wonder Woman would risk her life in order to achieve perfection!

WONDER WOMAN AT HER CROWN:
AMBITIOUS AND ASSURED

Wonder Woman is dynamic, driven, and determined. She's motivated by success and achievement and expects the best from herself and others. She rarely cracks under pressure. She embodies feminine strength, courage, and resilience. She's self-motivated, a natural strategist, and has an extraordinary capacity to create. If you want something done well, give it to a Wonder Woman.

Although she isn't indifferent to fashion or her looks, being pretty isn't enough for Wonder Woman; she wants to be known as a woman of substance and depth. More than any other archetype, Wonder Woman believes that she can accomplish anything she sets her mind to. Her personal history has confirmed this: studying hard meant top of the class; training hard meant winning; consistent practice meant being a virtuoso. Wonder Woman wants to leave a legacy. She wants beauty, brains, the perfect marriage, and perfect children. She wants to be remembered. She wants to have it all.

Wonder Woman measures her success by her environment and social structure. A New York–based Wonder Woman may be determined to be the head of a publishing company before the age of forty. A San Francisco–based Wonder Woman may strive to be the president of a successful tech start-up before she turns thirty. A Los Angeles–based actress won't be content starring in the film; she'll want to produce and direct it, too! If she lives in a small town, Wonder Woman wants to be on the board of the area's largest employer. She wants to be the biggest fish no matter the size of the pond.

Although many Wonder Women gravitate toward high-powered jobs, they don't have to work to identify with this archetype. A stay-at-home mom can be a Wonder Woman. She'll be the one directing her kids to take piano and French lessons, making sure her home always looks immaculate, and running a successful mommy-and-me blog. She prides herself on being busy and excelling at whatever she does.

Celebrated Wonder Women include Hillary Clinton, Sheryl Sandberg, Gwyneth Paltrow, Angelina Jolie, Gretchen Rubin, Jane Goodall, Miranda Priestly from *The Devil Wears Prada*, and your sister who just made partner at her law firm and has two children under the age of three.

THE BELIEF SYSTEM: "I AM WORTHY BECAUSE OF WHAT I DO"

When Wonder Woman is recognized for her excellence, she exudes charm, grace, and self-assurance. But if her work is disparaged, she can feel threatened, as if her whole life is under attack. Other archetypes simply accept the feedback and move on, but, for Wonder Woman, the pain can last for days or even longer. When this happens frequently, Wonder Woman may withdraw and shield herself from criticism by declining opportunities for exposure. She fears being wrong, as it makes her feel like a fraud, an imposter, a failure. This is devastating for a Wonder Woman, who prides herself on getting things right.

Wonder Woman will work until midnight for weeks (or years) to ensure her project, design, or speech is flawless, whereas the Femme Fatale or Ethereal will be happy with what they were able to get done in the time allocated. The Nurturer will only work long hours if it doesn't cause her to neglect her obligations to family or friends.

As Wonder Woman has been programmed to be the best, she can sacrifice her self-care and intimate relationships in the pursuit of excellence.

In her aptly titled book, *Wonder Women: Sex, Power, and the Quest for Perfection*, Barnard College president and author Debora Spar wrote, "Because we could do anything, we felt as if we had to do everything. . . . We'd convinced ourselves that having it all meant doing it all. Want to do well? Work hard. Want a nice dollhouse? Build it."[1]

If Wonder Woman is a stay-at-home mom, she must keep her mind intellectually stimulated so she feels she has a purpose. If not, she can become obsessed with her body, embracing the traits of a dysfunctional Femme Fatale. Two-hour daily training sessions and a fixation on her nonexistent imperfections become the norm. Her active mind becomes dull and she may ultimately live a lackluster existence, even if it's wrapped up in the opulence of a Park Avenue penthouse.

When I was working in finance in the early 2000s, I wanted to be just like the company's chief operating officer (COO). Three days after giving birth, this Wonder Woman was back running European operations. At the time, I perceived this poised woman, a mother and a corporate power-house, as the pinnacle of success who embodied my belief that a woman could have it all.

But years later, after a decade of consulting with countless Wonder Women like my COO, the illusion had shattered. I realized that far too many of these women were living in an underworld where joy was buried under the expectation of everything they thought they needed to be and do. Wonder Woman was stretched to depletion and her mind hijacked by a never-ending to-do list. So how did this otherwise accomplished arche-type wind up following this distorted script?

CHILDHOOD PATTERNS: FROM WONDER GIRLS TO WONDER WOMEN

The post-feminist movement ushered in herds of Wonder Women. Girls were encouraged to pursue careers as doctors, lawyers, bankers, or tech entrepreneurs, options that had eluded women of previous generations. Fathers wanted their daughters to excel and mothers wanted them to know that they could be anything they wanted to be. Good grades were the ticket to freedom, and Wonder Girls were praised for their scholastic accomplishments. They quickly learned that the more they did, the more attention they received. Straight As, swim team captain, and running the school newspaper—the Wonder Girl did it all. While these accolades boosted her self-confidence, she unwittingly tied her value to her ability. She created the subconscious imprint of "I am worthy because of what I do."

And American culture backed it up. Wonder Girl learned to be a busy girl. Idle time was perceived as wasted time. Her mother had banished

Barbie from the house because she feared sending her daughter the wrong message about female beauty. Instead, Mommy sent Wonder Girl to after-school karate and French lessons. Daddy wanted her to be a CEO, so he brought her books and encouraged her to do well in math. Future Wonder Woman was too busy to have playtime, a habit she proudly continued into adulthood. Being busy meant she was important.

Or perhaps it wasn't parents or society pushing her to succeed and showering her with opportunity; she may have grown up without material wealth and vowed to make her own way in the world. When my client Kayla was an impressionable twelve–year-old, she watched her mother's self-worth disintegrate along with her marriage and finances. Kayla could feel her mother's humiliation as she cleaned hotel rooms to make ends meet. Kayla unconsciously made the decision to become financially successful in order to avoid the feelings of shame she saw her mother endure. She sacrificed playtime for study time. She pursued excellence and intellect and is now one of the most prominent women in technology. But this success came at a cost, as it does for all Wonder Women.

When my parents divorced, my mother raised her four children mostly on her own. While she taught us impeccable manners and made us walk with books on our head so we had good posture, she felt embarrassed that she was not married and money was tight. I promised myself that I would never put myself in a position where I would depend on someone else for financial support. I had already internalized the belief that, since I would never be the prettiest, I would have to gain attention in another way, and I did so by being a smart student and overachiever. This pattern only intensified when my father praised me for receiving good grades or quizzed me on what I had learned in school. Witnessing my mother's sense of failure in tandem with the attention I got from my father for achieving firmly cemented my view that being smart was the path to acceptance.

WONDER GIRLS AND STRESS

I worry that many teenage girls are headed toward burnout. I've seen many sixteen-year-olds whose adrenal glands are working overtime. They have no energy, their periods are erratic, they're irritable, and they're sleeping fewer than six hours per night. They are Wonder Women–in-waiting. These girls are typically straight-A students, have track and field practice after school, work a part-time job, are auditioning for the lead in the school play, and always want to look beautiful on social media. It's too much for an adult woman to handle, let alone a developing one. We all need time for play, particularly teenagers.

If you know a young woman heading down this road, observe how she is valuing herself. Does she need to be reassured that she will still be respected, loved, and accepted if she's not the best at everything? You might also want to take her through the exercises to heal the mind in Part III. If she gets sick, depressed, or paralyzed by stress, she'll compromise her long-term goals, from college to career, and potentially miss out on simply having fun and being young. Most of all, be an inspiration for her—slow down, be graceful, and show her how it's done.

OUT OF BALANCE: "GET OUT OF MY WAY"

As with all of the archetypes, when Wonder Women are out of balance, there is both an amplification and a withdrawal of their traits. The amplification will present itself in the excessive pursuit of recognition. As Wonder Woman is programmed to believe that success is linear, the more effort she exerts, the greater the reward she expects. Sleep is cut back to an unsustainable six hours a night or less. She skips meals and can't remember the last time she cooked. Sex becomes nonexistent, which makes her feel even worse, as now she's not even a good lover!

In the amplification, Wonder Woman is a blur of activity moving with intensity from one to-do list item to the next. As time is her most precious resource, be prepared for Wonder Woman's fury when anyone slows her down. It's not that she is angry; it's simply that her schedule is so tight that any disruption means less time for her. Held up in traffic for twenty minutes? That could have been an extra twenty minutes of sleep. A meeting that ran over by fifteen minutes? That's when she planned to eat, so now she has to skip lunch. She's starving . . . and not just for food.

In fact, a nagging emptiness plagues far too many Wonder Women. I speculate that this comes in part from her de-prioritizing the human need for affection and attention and overvaluing her need for acknowledgment and appreciation. Recently, a fifty-eight-year-old Wonder Woman client of mine declared that she wanted a part-time boyfriend because her career demanded so much from her. This statement made me pause. We all, men and women, have an innate desire to connect on an emotional level. Real love is not needy or, as Wonder Woman fears, too soft or vulnerable. Professional achievement, no matter how successful you are, will never replace the aphrodisiac of real love.

Even if Wonder Woman has "settled down" into a long-term relationship, she must have something to keep her always-active mind engaged. I've seen too many Wonder Women in a loving marriage with children they adore who nonetheless find themselves asking, "Is this it?" A Nurturer or Femme Fatale may be content with this life, but not the Wonder Woman. She needs to accomplish things, otherwise she will feel depleted and she can end up resenting her partner or children for taking her away from something else that gives her independence and relevance.

Since Wonder Woman is so action-oriented, she usually acts in the amplification when she is out of balance. However, certain situations can cause her to withdraw and operate from a place of insecurity. When this happens, she is not the robust, strong, feminine force she likes to be but, rather, paralyzed into inaction for fear of criticism and humiliation. Due to one of my own childhood wounds, I would often decline opportunities to speak to large audiences. The fear of being wrong and considered a fraud was so powerful that I would instinctively say no to these opportunities. Once I altered this false belief, I jumped at every opportunity to speak and share my message.

THE WONDER WOMAN ARCHETYPE: THIRD CHAKRA

Wonder Woman is governed by her third chakra, which represents personal power. Strip her of her success (her education, career, money, smart kids, social status, or whatever she holds in high regard) and she'll feel a dull ache between her sternum and her belly button. This is where the third chakra is located. Wonder Woman will quickly want to get rid of this uncomfortable thought (or not even consider it!).

The third chakra is expressed through the color yellow. Any time Wonder Woman feels uncomfortable, she can support herself with the yellow color spectrum. She can skew her diet toward yellow foods such as pineapple, yellow bell peppers, yellow squash, golden beets, yellow tomatoes, yellow watermelon, and lemons. (Not yellow M&M's, Wonder Woman!) She can also wear yellow lingerie or use a swipe of golden eye shadow. In fact, she can add a dash of yellow or gold anywhere.

EATING BEHAVIOR: "I DESERVE IT!"

A Wonder Woman at her crown has a peaceful relationship with food. You instinctively know what to eat for your body and mood and don't feel the need to control—or be overly indulgent. You trust how food nourishes you, and if you gain some weight, you know precisely what to do to bring your diet back into balance.

However, when your crown is knocked off, you justify your daily consumption of dark chocolate (or a glass of red wine) by pointing to its antioxidant content (isn't it good for you?) and the fact that you deserve it. After all, you've had a hard day. You can also be a mindless eater, tossing M&M's into your mouth as you move from one meeting to the next. You skip meals, unintentionally, as your day can become so chaotic that you don't have time to take a break to eat. One Wonder Woman client refused to drink water during the day because she felt she didn't have time to make trips to the bathroom!

Wonder Woman can also adopt an all-or-nothing attitude regarding food. You're either on a diet or you've blown it, so all bets are off. You're eating raw salads—or shoving cookies into your mouth. Clients like these often say, "Just tell me what to do, and I'll do it," and they mean it in all sincerity. But while the intention is there, an invalidation from your boss, a sick child, or a nasty comment on social media can send you into a tailspin, and before you're even consciously aware of it, that leftover brownie you managed to avoid in the afternoon meeting has made its way into your mouth. Depending on how self-aware you are, the behavior will either stop there or you'll continue to eat mindlessly until you're disappointed enough to start a "detox" the next day.

THE CHALLENGE FOR WONDER WOMAN: IT'S OKAY TO NOT BE BUSY

Wonder Woman has internalized the misguided belief that success equals recognition, and recognition means you're important and therefore worthy of attention. From this, you have created your protective (but cracking) veneer of busyness, perfection, and control. But as you know (or will soon discover), this is a destructive fallacy, an illusion that can lead to physical imbalances such as fatigue, a bloated belly, and anxiety. It's also left you with an emptiness that ever-so-quietly whispers, "Something is wrong." The only thing that's wrong, of course, is your erroneous belief that you are valued for your successes. You're not. You are valued for who you are—flaws and all.

If you want to have it all, you can, but you can't expect to be the best mother, the best lover, and the best worker with godlike intuitive powers all at the same time! You can, however, be the most *balanced* mother, lover, and worker with godlike intuitive powers. While this sounds less impressive than "being the best," this shift will enable you to be sexier, softer, and more at ease. It will lead to a richer life, not a perfect life. Ironically, that richness is what you thought a perfect life would give you.

No archetype will find the deconstruction of her self-worth matrix easy. Like footprints in concrete, the old mind-set appears irreversible, but just as fresh concrete can be poured to erase the old footprints, new thoughts can be formed to replace old ones. When you stop defining other people by their accomplishments, you will find it easier to do the same for yourself. The first mini-challenge for Wonder Woman is to go to a party and *not* ask someone what they do for a living. Instead, try asking them what they do for pleasure. It's adding a little Femme Fatale oomph to your life.

To wear your crown as a Wonder Woman, you must remember the unique power of your feminine energies—tenderness, warmth, compassion, intuition, and empathy. You must realize that a soft heart doesn't mean a soft head. You must embrace the idea that strength and kindness can coexist, as can being smart and sensual. You can also learn from the other archetypes to help you ascend to the crown.

- You can embody the Femme Fatale to engage in the sensual pleasures in life—like savoring a sweet rose tea on the sofa while wrapped in a soft blanket.
- You can tap into your inner Ethereal to access your intuition and blend it with your intellect for clarity, truth, and wisdom.
- You can learn from the Nurturer how to open your heart and live from a place of deep connection and trust.

When you add the positive attributes of the other archetypes, you rise up to the crown to transform yourself from a woman of importance to a woman of inspiration, elegance, and grace.

THE WONDER WOMAN FOOD PRESCRIPTION

In order to support your transition to a whole woman, you need to address the hormonal imbalances that your Wonder Woman lifestyle has triggered. Emotional and physical stressors cause a surge in the stress-coping hormones adrenaline, noradrenaline, and cortisol. At the right level, these hormones are fat burners. At the wrong level, they inhibit fat burning. What's more, excess cortisol tells the body to store fat around the abdominal area, and this is why chronically stressed Wonder Women put weight on their belly first. (On a side note, most belly-busting supplements are just cortisol regulators.)

HORMONAL IMBALANCE: CORTISOL AND BEYOND

Wonder Woman's dominant hormone is cortisol. When your body is in balance, cortisol levels should rise when stressors are encountered and then return to normal when the stressors have gone away. But if you are constantly bombarded with trivial stressors—two hundred unanswered emails, kids drawing on walls with permanent makers, or an error on a report—your stress hormones can remain elevated and start to interfere with other hormones. Excess cortisol can also impair liver function and slow the removal of toxins and excess hormones from the body, contributing to fatigue, weight gain, skin breakouts, and hormonal imbalances.

One hormone that cortisol affects is the thyroid hormone thyroxine (T4). Since thyroxine revs up the body (and so does cortisol), if your cortisol levels are elevated, your brain will tell the thyroid to produce less T4 to slow you down. When this happens, you can feel wired and tired at the same time. Your cortisol is elevated, keeping you awake and alert, but your metabolism has declined. If you catch this early enough, all you need to do is decrease the cortisol response and the thyroid will auto-correct. But if you don't, then you'll need to restore both your adrenal and thyroid function. I have specifically designed the Wonder Woman's diet to restore both her adrenals and thyroid. I've also included supplements at the end of this chapter to help with the reset.

Cortisol also affects the production of progesterone, one of the sex hormones, which balances excess estrogen and aids cognition. Cortisol and progesterone are made from the same precursor, and the body will prioritize the synthesis of cortisol over progesterone. That's because progesterone is, among other things, the pregnancy hormone, and the body does not prioritize fertility when under stress. It wants you to escape a stressful situation so it will give you more cortisol to help you out. If you're a Wonder Woman with PMS, hot flashes, or brain fogginess, it's highly likely that you have low progesterone. The solution, however, isn't necessarily to add more progesterone, it's to calm down cortisol and reinterpret the stressors so that the body can create more progesterone naturally.

ADRENAL FATIGUE—LOW STRESS HORMONES

Over time, if the stressors are not removed or reinterpreted, the brain's communication with the adrenal glands starts to falter. The adrenals produce less and less cortisol, adrenaline, and noradrenaline, making it difficult for you to deal with stressful situations. Where you once had too-high levels of stress hormones in your body, you now have too little. This is known as adrenal fatigue, and the symptoms associated with it—chronic fatigue, depression, decreased libido, weight loss resistance—are what we commonly refer to as "burnout." You have stressed your body beyond the breaking point and now struggle to deal with even the most minor stress.

What's more, too little cortisol also impacts the body's ability to convert T4 to the active thyroid hormone, triiodothyronine (T3), which regulates energy and boosts the metabolism. If your metabolism is not functioning properly, you will put on weight more easily and find it more difficult to lose it. In essence, when you have too little cortisol, it becomes more difficult for you to lose weight, even while on a diet. This is why it's essential that you 1) add in the supplements that improve cortisol regulation, and 2) work through Part III, "The Six Rs to Heal Your Mind," to change the beliefs and behaviors that add stress to your life. If you can't get out of bed without a cup of coffee nearby, feel exhausted after even a moderate amount of exercise, or find yourself nodding off at work in the middle of the day, then it's highly likely you are adrenally fatigued. If this is the case, it's even more important not to skip meals and eat every three hours so that the adrenals are not calling on your scant supply of stress hormones to stabilize your blood-sugar levels. I highly recommend you skip coffee, intermittent fasting, restrictive diets, and high-intensity exercise. Instead, get nine hours of sleep, meditate, and eat the nourishing diet prescribed for Wonder Woman. The body will recover; you just need to give it the tools and nutrients to do so.

THE COPING MECHANISM

Wonder Woman eats (and drinks) as a way to switch her brain off. If your habit is a nightly glass of wine, you're unlikely to go back to your emails when you're a little tipsy. The wine gives you permission to check out. You might also decompress from a stressful day with half a bar of dark chocolate while listening to a podcast. Whatever your choice of distraction, you are rewarding yourself for making it through a chaotic day. If you're an out-of-balance Wonder Woman, this "treat" can be the only thing that brings you joy, and you'll be resistant to giving it up. However, as you add more joy into other aspects of your life your desire for these treats will diminish. And by recognizing this habit for what it is—permission to switch off—you can simply allow yourself to do so without guilt. Remember, the goal is to be a layered, complex woman who alchemizes all of the positive attributes of all four archetypes (sensuality, compassion, intuition, and intellect), not just a woman who works, and that requires investment into each of these four areas.

WONDER WOMAN'S MEAL PLAN

As Wonder Women are always on the go, I have found that following a food formula is often easier for her than sticking to a specific ten-day plan. As such, I have outlined the guidelines below so that you can apply them anywhere—at home, at restaurants, or while traveling. To make these concepts more tangible, I've included a ten-day meal plan in

Chapter 13, but remember: you do not need to follow the ten-day meal plan to the letter, just get the concept right.

Step 1: Improve Your Daily Eating Regimen

1. Start each morning with an elixir to bring your feminine energy into balance: add 1 teaspoon of rose water to 4 ounces of cool filtered water.

2. Always eat a protein-based breakfast: no oats, fruit, or green vegetable juice.

3. Be sure lunch and dinner each consist of seven ingredients: three vegetables, one protein, two fats, and one carb. These meals should look like the food plate on page 53.

4. Remember the Rule of 4 when it comes to portion size: a portion equals 4 ounces of protein, ¼ avocado (or other fats), ¼ cup of carbs, and up to 4 cups of vegetables.

5. Don't skip your four p.m. snack. If you do, you'll come home starving and will want to shove whatever food you can find into your mouth. At four p.m., take ten minutes to decompress, make yourself a tea, or drink the adrenal tonic below and eat a nutrient-dense snack, making sure the number of calories in the snack is no greater than your ideal weight in pounds.

6. In the evening, wind down with Wonder Woman's tea, which is specifically designed to support adrenal function and promote liver detoxification.

Step 2: Choose the Right Foods

Specific foods can help to rebalance the Wonder Woman's physical and emotional state. Add the suggestions below to your daily eating regimen. Remember, subtle tweaks can make a big difference.

1. Eat bitter vegetables daily. This includes arugula, broccoli rabe, dandelion greens, endive, radicchio, escarole, watercress, mustard greens, and kale. Bitter vegetables stimulate liver detoxification and support adrenal function. Enjoy a watercress soup or snack on endive with hummus.

2. Add yellow fruit or vegetables. This helps align the third chakra to improve feelings of self-worth and self-confidence. Try yellow bell peppers in a salad or pineapple as an afternoon snack.

3. Eat 4 ounces of clean animal protein at lunch and dinner. Do not eat more than this unless you want to build muscle. Choose a variety of proteins, not just chicken because it's convenient. Eat seafood at least four times a week for its selenium and iodine to support the thyroid. Organic tofu and tempeh can be consumed once a week but not more than that because of their weak estrogenic effect. (Wonder Woman can have estrogen dominance due to low progesterone levels.)

4. Eat grass-fed red meat once a week. Red meat is rich in iron and zinc, which help support Wonder Woman's energy levels. Don't exclude red meat because you've read that it's "bad" or that it increases cholesterol levels. If you're eating 12 ounces of steak a day with fries, then it's an issue, but 4 ounces once a week is just fine. Try organic lamb cutlets with chimichurri sauce or organic steak served with Dijon mustard.

5. Eat ¼ cup of starchy carbs at lunch and dinner. Wonder Women are not as sensitive to carbohydrates as Nurturers and will often feel more balanced when they add a hint of carbs to their meals. This amount is equivalent to 4 tablespoons. It is a sprinkling. Since it's a relatively small quantity, stick with one type of starchy carb per meal: beans *or* rice, not beans *and* rice. If you skip the carbs at lunch, this is not license to double them at dinner, as more carbs will cause a bigger spike in insulin levels.

6. Use nuts and seeds to your energetic advantage. If you are feeling scattered, eat more nuts as they help to ground you. Snack on almond crackers with avocado or add cashews to wok-tossed vegetables. If you are feeling overwhelmed, opt for seeds as they are energetically and chemically lighter. Snack on turmeric-spiced pumpkin seeds or add hemp seeds to salads.

7. Make your snacks work for you by eating snacks that support your adrenals and thyroid. It's best not to eat gluten-free pretzels or popcorn, which don't do anything other than keep your fingers busy. Instead, eat snacks that are rich in magnesium, vitamin C, omega-3s, zinc, selenium, and iodine. Try the adrenal tonic (recipe below), turmeric hemp milk lattes, green vegetable juices, nori with ¼ avocado, 4 Brazil nuts with goji berries, fresh figs, or home-roasted sunflower seeds with sea salt.

8. Avoid gluten and dairy. All archetypes need to avoid gluten and dairy for the first four weeks of their new diet, but this is even more imperative for Wonder Woman. If you eat foods that you are sensitive to, you will inflame your body, calling on cortisol to dampen the inflammation.

9. Be generous with fresh herbs. Add basil, cilantro, dill, and parsley to salads. These herbs help to bind up toxins, making it easier for the liver to remove them from the body.

Foods that rebalance the Wonder Woman: grilled fish, organic poultry, raw salads, cooked vegetables, fresh herbs, bitter vegetables, yellow fruits and vegetables, nuts, seeds, and a small amount of red meat, grains, legumes, and starchy vegetables.

Foods that should be kept to a minimum: dairy, gluten, soy, and sweets.

THE WONDER WOMAN ADRENAL TONIC

If you have been feeling fatigued, anxious, or depressed, your adrenals probably aren't functioning as well as they should. Adding this tonic to your daily repertoire can help to restore their function. If you are adrenally fatigued, add the licorice root as specified in the recipe.

¼ teaspoon powdered ashwagandha root
½ teaspoon powdered rhodiola
½ teaspoon powdered cordyceps
1 teaspoon coconut sugar
1 teaspoon raw cacao
1 teaspoon coconut oil
Dash of cinnamon and nutmeg
*1 cup nut or seed milk such as almond or flax, or coconut milk
    (heated or not)*
*If adrenally fatigued, add ⅛ teaspoon of powdered licorice
    root; otherwise skip*

Place all ingredients in a blender, cover, and blend until well mixed. Serve either warm or over ice. If you've added the licorice root because of adrenal fatigue, and you find it too overpowering, add an additional teaspoon of cacao and coconut oil. You could also add these ingredients to your morning smoothie instead of drinking them as a tonic.

All of the active ingredients in the tonic have consistently been shown to improve adrenal function. (Cacao, coconut sugar, and the spices are primarily for taste.) Ashwagandha increases brain-derived neurotrophic factor (BDNF), which stimulates brain cell renewal.[2] It also improves energy levels and mitochondrial health.[3] Rhodiola increases cognitive function, attention, mental acuity, and clarity. It also improves stress resistance by increasing a "stress-sensor" protein.[4] Cordyceps are medicinal mushrooms that improve physical and mental stamina as well as boost the libido.[5] They also increase natural killer cells to fight off bacteria and viruses.[6] Licorice root mimics the effect of cortisol, so add if you are adrenally fatigued.[7] Do not add licorice root if you have high cortisol or high blood pressure, as licorice root can increase both. All ingredients can be purchased online and I have created this adrenal tonic already blended for ease of use. More information can be found in Resources.

THE WONDER WOMAN TEA

This tea unites the femininity of rose with the masculinity of holy basil to decrease adrenal fatigue and anxiety. It's blended with nettle and cardamom to support liver detoxification. The recipe below makes a single 12-ounce serving, but you can make the tea blend in larger quantities and store it in an airtight canister.

  2 teaspoons holy basil
  2 teaspoons nettle
  4 dried rosebuds
  4 cardamom pods

Combine the ingredients in a small pot with 12 ounces of hot water. Steep for 5 minutes, then strain into a tea cup. Add more hot water if the tea is too strong.

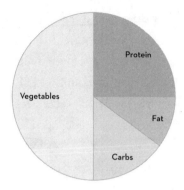

THE WONDER WOMAN'S FOOD PLATE

Step 3: Supplement Strategically

In addition to the adrenal tonic, add in some foundational supplements to support the adrenals and thyroid.

- **Vitamin C:** More vitamin C is stored in the adrenal glands than anywhere else in the body.[8] The body needs vitamin C to synthesize cortisol and adrenaline as well as the pleasure neurotransmitter dopamine. Vitamin C also helps to regulate bowel movements. Take 1,000 mg per day.
- **B Complex:** Take an activated B complex to help boost energy levels and regulate sex hormone levels. It also helps to metabolize alcohol. Look for the activated forms such as L-5-MTHF (folate), pyridoxine HCl (B6), and methylcobalamin (B12). Take one daily after food; two on the days you drink alcohol.
- **Magnesium:** Magnesium is a natural relaxant. Take 300 mg of magnesium glycinate (or magnesium citrate if constipated) before bed as magnesium also helps encourage a deeper level of sleep.
- **Phosphatidylserine (PS):** This helps protect cortisol from damaging neurons in the hippocampus, where your long-term memory is stored. Take 200 mg before bed.

- **5-HTP:** If you can't sleep due to excess cortisol, add 50 mg 5-HTP daily before bed. This is the precursor to serotonin and melatonin. If you're taking a selective serotonin reuptake inhibitor (SSRI), speak to your physician before taking 5-HTP.
- **EPA/DHA (omega-3):** If you don't eat oily fish like wild salmon and halibut four times a week, take 1,000 mg of this omega-3 supplement daily. This helps sensitize the receptors to the stress hormones and rebuild the hippocampus, which is damaged by long-term exposure to cortisol.
- **Thyroid-Supporting Supplement:** If needed, take a thyroid supplement that contains iodine, selenium, zinc, and tyrosine to help support thyroid levels.

As you ascend to the crown and rebalance your physical body, you can loosen up on these guidelines. You can increase your carbohydrate portion to ½ cup per meal at breakfast, lunch, and dinner. You can also substitute one of your lunches or dinners for a vegan meal and include up to ¾ cup of protein-rich carbs such as lentils, chickpeas, and quinoa instead of animal protein. If you find your weight stagnating, you should return to the baseline program outlined above.

EXERCISE SOLUTIONS FOR WONDER WOMAN

Wonder Women benefit from a combination of high-intensity classes to burn off that excess adrenaline (unless they're adrenally fatigued, in which case take yoga or Pilates classes four times a week) as well as some light to medium weight training. Ideal types of exercise include rebounding, sprints, jumping rope, boxing, HIIT, plyometrics, circuit training, dancing, and biking. Try any combination of these four times a week and take a yoga class once a week. If using weights, opt for small-to-medium weights but target a high rep count to help tone and shape your muscles. If you want to build muscle mass, do fewer reps with more weight.

CHAPTER 4

The Femme Fatale

―――

With her long, luscious locks and deep emerald eyes, Sara captivates both men and women, but beneath her alluring facade she is deeply scared; scared to gain weight and scared to age. She is ashamed that she thinks about her physical appearance as much as she does, but she doesn't know how to stop it. Even when she was at her ideal weight, she wasn't able to enjoy it because she was so fearful that an extra bite of dessert would immediately make her gain back her weight and all of the sadness and insecurity that accompanied it. At times, she feels imprisoned by this body obsession and wants nothing more than to be free of it. She wants to be radiant and magnetic and would do anything to get there . . . other than eat more food.

Sara is a Femme Fatale, but an out-of-balance one. She can either ascend to the crown by uncoupling her self-worth from her physical appearance or she can allow her perception of her looks to continue to threaten her sense of self. Almost every Femme Fatale will face this crossroad at some point in her life.

THE FEMME FATALE AT HER CROWN: BEAUTIFUL AND BEGUILING

When the Femme Fatale feels secure in her beauty, she is mesmerizing. She is sensual, alluring, playful, and passionate, and you can't help but notice her. She's the one throwing her head back and laughing with joy at the silliest things. You'll find her sipping tea and giggling with her girlfriends at a French tea salon or curled up on the sofa in a cashmere throw, reading a juicy novel. The provocative photography of Helmut Newton, Herb Ritts, and Ellen Von Unwerth captures the essence of the Femme Fatale in balance: strong, powerful, and sexy. When the Femme Fatale wears her crown, she draws beauty and people into her life with ease. Her presence encourages other women to lead a more resplendent life. It's "I'll have what she is having." But when the Femme Fatale doesn't feel beautiful, it's a very different story.

Celebrated Femme Fatales include Elizabeth Taylor, Demi Moore, Sharon Stone, Kim Kardashian, the Bond Girls, Lana del Rey, Julia Roberts in *Pretty Woman*, Manet's *Olympia*, and that gorgeous Parisian woman whom you (and your partner) were captivated by.

THE BELIEF SYSTEM: "BEAUTY GETS YOU WHAT YOU WANT"

Because the Femme Fatale's power source is her physical appearance, her sense of self tends to rise and fall with the average beauty quotient in the room. If she's the prettiest, she'll feel more confident. If she's not, she'll feel less than. When she's at her crown, she knows she has more to offer than just physical appearance. But when she isn't at her crown, a hint of cellulite, a pinch of fat, a chipped nail, or a new wrinkle can throw her into complete panic. She can become fixated on her imperfections. This anxiety might last for a minute or it can be the dark tunnel in which she lives every day of her life. To the outside observer, her flaws (if you even noticed them) are minor. But in her mind, a flaw, no matter how inconsequential, is a mark against her value as a woman.

The dichotomy between a balanced Femme Fatale and an out-of-balance Femme Fatale is so striking that you'd be hard pressed to find a similarity between the two, but their underlying belief—that beauty is the trump card—binds them together. No other archetype has such polarity between the balance and imbalance. If you're a balanced Femme Fatale, the out-of-balance Femme Fatale may not resonate with you, but you can still appreciate the pain they experience; you just have more resilience and less need for validation.

We can't blame the Femme Fatale for buying into the warped notion that physical appearance dictates her worth. She has simply internalized society's fixation on beauty. We live in a culture that says the goodies in life are rationed. Love, sisterhood, kindness, time, romantic partners, money, and attention are the purview of the *best* people, which the Femme Fatale interprets as the *prettiest. Without good looks, you will miss out.* This kind of insecurity fuels the economy by enticing you to buy things to make you feel more attractive. And if you don't feel attractive, you blame yourself.

While the feminist movement of the '60s and '70s attacked the status quo that said a woman needed to attract a prosperous partner in order to have financial stability, the Femme Fatale continues to believe in this precarious paradigm, and that being attractive is the best way to achieve this goal. As Gloria Steinem says in *Revolution from Within*, "It was as if the female spirit were a garden that had grown beneath the shadows of the barriers for so long that it kept growing in the same pattern, even after some of the barriers were gone."[1]

Similarly, social media has morphed into a self-consciousness-inducing milieu where bikini-clad women have the most engagement. The message is, if you are pretty and fit, you can have an enviable life with influence. If you can't, you will spend your life on the sidelines never feeling good enough.

Wanting to look attractive doesn't necessarily mean you're a Femme Fatale. To be a Femme Fatale, you must derive your sense of self primarily from your physical attributes. There is nothing wrong with wanting to look more attractive; it is only damaging when it becomes the sole obsession in your life, something the Femme Fatale is prone to.

THE FEMME FATALE ARCHETYPE: THE SECOND CHAKRA

The second chakra has a stranglehold on the Femme Fatale. It represents pleasure and how others perceive you and reflects the emotions connected to sex and power. An out-of-balance second chakra can lead to social withdrawal or to overexposure as a way to seek validation from others. It is located in the pelvic area and includes the reproductive organs. It's not surprising that Femme Fatales can use seduction to get their way—or shut it down when they feel unattractive.

The second chakra is represented by the color orange. When the Femme Fatale feels overly controlling or judgmental (toward herself or others), she can bolster her diet with orange foods such as papaya, peaches, apricots, nectarines, orange bell peppers, butternut squash, and sweet potatoes. She can carry an orange purse or wear orange lingerie to help strengthen her sense of self. The orange spectrum helps to rebalance a weak second chakra.

THE CHILDHOOD PATTERNS: FROM BEAST TO BEAUTY

Every Femme Fatale I have worked with became that archetype as the result of an upsetting childhood memory. She did not become a Femme Fatale in response to constant praise and adoration of her looks; she used her looks strategically to cope with a lack of attention in her life. Marilyn Monroe, one of the world's best-known sex symbols, spent much of her childhood in foster homes when her mother was committed to a psychiatric hospital. From an early age she learned that seduction could bring her attention, which became a proxy for the affection and approval that was missing in her life. She became the Femme Fatale.

One client oscillated between restriction and binge eating for more than three decades. When she was ten, her handsome father left her two-hundred-pound mother for a ballerina. She learned to restrict her food, believing that being skinny was how you kept a man, but would binge-eat to rebel against this belief and unconsciously offer support to her mother, who never recovered emotionally after losing her husband.

Other Femme Fatales have taken derogatory comments about their weight or looks to heart. One client was told by her eye doctor at the age of fourteen that she would never be a model because her eyes were not symmetrical. This sent her into a binge-and-purge routine for over a decade, believing that if she had a "hot body" people wouldn't notice the flaw in her facial structure. Whatever the memory, for the Femme Fatale it has created the imprint that beauty is power and if you aren't beautiful then life will be wretched and miserable.

If you're a mother and are worried about complimenting your daughter on her looks because you don't want her to value herself on her physical appearance, please don't be. I've had Wonder Women in my practice who have cried because their parents *only* gave them accolades for their academic achievements and not for their looks. They felt unattractive because they were never given compliments on their looks, and today they and still carry that scar. Until our culture stops overvaluing physical appearance, women will be subject to criticism—by themselves or others—for the way they look. Making sure your daughter knows she's beautiful, and helping her *believe* it, will shield her from society's judgment. We need our girls to feel whole, and that means positive affirmations for the physical, emotional, intuitive, *and* intellectual.

OUT OF BALANCE: "I LOOK FAT . . . I LOOK HOT . . . I LOOK FAT . . . I LOOK HOT . . ."

When your self-worth is based on your looks, you'll instinctively seek out things that make you look more attractive, but this is where things can go haywire. An aging Femme Fatale can have too much facial surgery in an attempt to retain her beauty. Playboy Playmates, Real Housewives, and bikini-clad girls posting selfies on yachts are caricatures of out-of-balance Femme Fatales seeking validation from outsiders instead of believing that they are already beautiful.

Similarly, an out-of-balance Femme Fatale can use sex to feel worthy. My client Jessica finally felt visible when she learned to use seduction and sex as a tool for attention. Tragically, this behavior left her feeling emptier and hollower than before. Her weight would go up and down—along with her self-worth—as she used food to suppress her feelings of disconnection and loneliness. It was only when she healed her childhood scars of neglect and came to believe she was worthy of love because of who she is, not her sexuality, that she was finally able to restore her self-worth and heal the depression that had persisted for most of her life.

The Femme Fatale is also the most likely to make snarky remarks about another woman's weight and clothing. She'll ask, "Doesn't that woman have any respect for herself? How can she be wolfing down that pizza?" Or "Please tell me I don't look like *that* when I wear my denim shorts." The sad part is, she is judging everyone else because she is afraid of receiving the same judgment herself. She's held in the bondage of her own tongue, projecting her own insecurities onto others.

These examples are the Femme Fatale in amplification. Her natural sensuality and playfulness have become exaggerated, unhealthy, and at times abusive to herself and others. If you're not a Femme Fatale and find yourself rolling your eyes at her need for validation on her physical appearance, step back and offer some compassion. This is a coping strategy she uses to feel better about herself, just as Wonder Woman works seventy hours a week and the Nurturer does everything for everyone. It's not vacuous or superficial (as many people perceive it to be); it's a way to protect her value. She's fearful that when her physical appeal diminishes, she'll be discarded like a broken toy.

The Femme Fatale can also exhibit mild delusions. After eating a food that she perceives as "bad," she will swear that she can "see" it on herself immediately even though it's impossible for fat to be created that quickly. My client Louise ate a second piece of pie with ice cream one evening and she was absolutely certain that she had gained extra body fat right in that moment. The next day, she didn't want to go to the beach, even though just one weekend before she had felt lean and radiant, jumping around on the beach in a bikini, throwing a Frisbee, and paddle-boarding. Her friends finally convinced her to join them, but she went in a cover-up, fearful people would judge her for having put on weight. She later discovered that she had actually weighed *less* on that second weekend; her mind had played tricks on her because she felt guilty at having overeaten. The out-of-balance Femme Fatale doesn't want to suffer like this, but she doesn't know how to free herself from this obsession.

EATING BEHAVIOR:
"FOOD IS EITHER GOOD OR BAD"

When the Femme Fatale wears her crown, she enjoys the pleasure and sensuality of food. She's tactile and savors every morsel and chooses foods that naturally bring out her most feminine self.

If you're an out-of-balance Femme Fatale, however, you can be overly restrictive or binge-eat out of disgust with yourself. You worry that if you overeat, even once, you'll blow up like Violet from *Charlie and the Chocolate Factory*. Your behavior with food mirrors your obsession with your looks. You can become fixated on healthy food to the point of orthorexia, a pathological condition where you exclusively eat food you consider healthy (which may only be greens and whitefish). You may also exhibit anorexic tendencies as a technique of restraint and will applaud yourself for not eating. Eating disorders are more prevalent among Femme Fatales, though they are not exclusive to this archetype. Wonder Women, in their pursuit for perfection, can also engage in this behavior. So, too, can an Ethereal who loses herself and attempts to find acceptance by mimicking the Femme Fatale.

Sometimes the Femme Fatale's rigid attitudes about food can be the result of chronic digestive issues. If your belly gets distended after eating beans, grains, and cruciferous vegetables, you may declare them to be kryptonite and forever avoid these foods rather than investigating why they made your body react that way. If you insist on placing certain foods in the "bad" category, you'll ultimately deny yourself nutrient-rich foods that would contribute to your physical beauty. This is what happened with my client Stephanie. She'd previously been diagnosed with SIBO (small intestinal bacterial overgrowth), and part of the protocol for getting rid of the bacteria was to avoid all grains. She'd interpreted this to mean that she should avoid grains *for life*, not just during treatment. This became a convenient excuse for restricting what she ate. Behind this justification, she was fearful that just one taste of a carb would trigger an unstoppable binge. Her digestive issues legitimatized her disordered eating and took control of her mind.

On such a restrictive diet the Femme Fatale will, rightly, feel deprived—of food as well as pleasure elsewhere in her life. This can precipitate a binge episode. Once she starts, the guilt will become so unbearable that she'll often continue eating even more food in an attempt to punish herself. This may be anything from an extra apple (which is not on her rigid plan) or massive bowls of popcorn followed by dark chocolate and more. Guilt and shame are the drivers for the binge. The more shameful she feels about it, the more she'll end up eating.

Not surprisingly, the Femme Fatale can struggle socially with food unless surrounded by other Femme Fatales. She may cancel dinner dates because she don't trust herself to stop eating. If she does this often enough, she can become melancholic and depressed because connection and intimacy are vital for a woman's sanity.

THE CHALLENGE FOR THE FEMME FATALE: LEARNING TO GO DEEPER THAN SKIN-DEEP

Convincing yourself that beauty isn't currency is not an easy task, as you've viewed life through this superficial lens for as long as you can recall. But once you accept this, your self-worth will no longer be contingent on your appearance. That sinking feeling you experience when everyone in the room (or by the pool) appears more beautiful or skinnier than you will simply evaporate; it will no longer matter to you. While this may be hard for you to fathom, this is what freedom is. To reach this point, you will need to examine and reinterpret the memories that caused you to believe that your appearance determines your value.

As a Femme Fatale you are constantly judging your physical appearance against others', so your first mini-challenge is to create an "add-on" compliment. That means, when someone compliments you, you don't just say "thank you" or "this old thing," but instead extend the compliment by explaining how it makes you feel (and that feeling can only be positive!). For instance, if someone says, "You look so beautiful tonight," you can respond with, "Oh thank you, this dress makes me *feel* so amazing. It reminds me of summer and that makes me *feel* so good!" By doing this, you have responded from a place of feeling, not judgment. While the compliment was on your physical appearance, your response was not—it was on a positive feeling. You'll also notice how engaged the person complimenting you becomes when you respond in this way. By offering a bit of insight into yourself, you are creating a connection with someone that has nothing to do with your appearance but rather with your uplifting response.

Embodying the positive traits of the other archetypes is fundamental for the Femme Fatale's rise to the crown and to breaking your fixation with your physical appearance.

- It's essential that you awaken your spiritual self by embracing your inner Ethereal. By experiencing the power of her magnetic, energetic body, you can heal the scars that have caused you to excessively focus on your physical body.
- By embracing the Wonder Woman, you are reminded of your dignity and resilience. Your inner Wonder Woman can hold you strong when the feeling of being "not pretty enough" emerges and you want to retreat into isolation.
- The Nurturer can teach you compassion. As you soften your judgment of others, it will be mirrored with compassion toward yourself.

When you embody these traits, you will have a magnetic quality that is hard to resist. You will sparkle with pleasure and become a muse for women wanting to live a more sensual life.

THE FEMME FATALE FOOD PRESCRIPTION

Unlike Nurturers, Wonder Women, and Ethereals, whose archetypes usually corresponds to a particular body type, a Femme Fatale can take on any body type depending on her eating behavior. If you carry weight on your hips and thighs like a Nurturer but source your self-worth from your physical body, you are still a Femme Fatale, but one with elevated insulin and estrogen levels that are influencing where you store fat. If you store fat on your stomach like the Wonder Woman, then cortisol is your dominant hormone. If you look more like the Ethereal, then lower levels of estrogen may be shaping your body and contributing to symptoms of depression and amenorrhea.

HORMONAL IMBALANCES: DRIVEN BY BEHAVIORS

When you ascended to your crown, you are not preoccupied with your physical self. You are sensual, playful, and inspirational. You might be a voluptuous woman who brings to mind the Greek goddess Aphrodite, or you might be five pounds overweight because you love the sensuality of sharing a delicious meal and have no desire to change your social life.

If you are out of balance, however, you can resort to problematic eating behaviors that will naturally affect your body and biochemistry. If you are continually restricting food to fit into an itsy-bitsy bikini or using intermittent fasting in the hope of expediting weight loss, you can stress out your adrenals and cause a spike in your levels of the stress hormone cortisol. Elevated cortisol slows down the metabolism by impeding the production of the thyroid-regulating hormone thyroxine. Add this to the stress that you are already prone to feel about your body and you create a recipe for adrenal fatigue and hormonal imbalances, both of which can lead to weight gain. If this describes you, and you have been feeling burned out or fatigued, or if you tend to store fat in the belly area, read Chapter 3, "The Wonder Woman," to learn more about how adrenal function affects weight gain.

The Femme Fatale's restrictive eating can also trip an overeating backlash. You're hungry, frustrated, and irritable and can find yourself drowning in a sea of chocolate wrappers. The shame of overeating can lead to a perpetual shame-binge-restrict cycle. If this continues for long enough, your body will have trouble regulating its insulin and estrogen levels. When this happens, you will store weight all over your body, but particularly on your upper thighs, and your body will start to mimic the Nurturer's. (For more information about the biochemical reasons behind this weight gain, see Chapter 2, "The Nurturer.")

This may be hard for the Femme Fatale to swallow (no pun intended), but at a certain point, your body needs *more* calories if you want to lose weight. If you restrict food to the point that you are not getting enough calories, your body will take this as a signal that food has become scarce, and it will slow down your metabolism by changing the thyroid hormones to conserve energy. Specifically, it increases rT3 (reverse triiodothyronine), an inactive thyroid hormone that blocks the thyroid receptor cells from listening to T3, the active thyroid hormone. This is a double whammy: less T3 and less available thyroid receptor sites. Starving yourself simply makes the situation worse. To lose again, you may need to eat more calories, in particular carbohydrates, to reactive T3 and deactivate rT3. While this goes against current "calories in, calories out" logic, your body is not a robot. You're a complicated organism with protective mechanisms in place to stop you from starving and ultimately dying from lack of food. If this sounds like you, you may need to eat a little bit more like the Ethereal, with a higher level of carbohydrates, particularly if you exercise a lot.

While Femme Fatales should follow their food plate guidelines, they are notorious overachievers with their caloric restriction. It's imperative that you don't dip too low beneath your basal metabolic rate (BMR). Eating 800 calories for weeks on end will backfire. If you're not sure how much you should be eating, see the box below to determine your minimum daily calorie intake.

BASAL METABOLIC RATE

Your basal metabolic rate (BMR) refers to the minimum number of calories you need to consume daily in order for your body to function while at rest. Your BMR is determined by your height, weight, muscle, and age and is roughly equivalent to ten times your current weight. So if you weigh 130 pounds, you should eat roughly 1,300 calories per day, at minimum, for maintenance. For weight loss, subtract 200 calories. That means, your caloric intake should not dip below 1,100 calories. If you weigh 170 pounds, your BMR is around 1,700 per day, your caloric intake should not dip below 1,500 for weight loss. If you exercise, this number will increase since your body is burning more calories. As the Femme Fatale is prone to overexercising, it's important that she take her exercise into account when determining the minimum number of calories to eat.

EATING DISORDERS

Her tendency to restrict food intake makes the Femme Fatale the most prone of all of the archetypes to eating disorders. Perhaps you have learned that being skinny increases your confidence, and the more confident you are, the more attention you get, so you begin to restrict your calories in order to get the validation you crave. If this behavior turns into an eating disorder like anorexia or bulimia, which are fundamentally driven by disordered thinking rather than actual appearance, you may develop a subconscious desire *not* to resolve the disorder. Your disorder attracts attention, and you subconsciously worry that if you get healthy, you will lose the attention. Here again we see how the psychological is inextricably linked with the physical. If this is you, please seek out psychological assistance. Eating disorders rarely resolve themselves without professional intervention.

THE FEMME FATALE MEAL PLAN

The Femme Fatale's plan closely mimics the macronutrient composition laid out for the Wonder Woman, but there are subtle differences between the two, and these differences speak to the Femme Fatale's mind-set. The guidelines below will restore balance to the body and improve your ability to lose weight healthily, regardless of your body type. Let go of the notion that restricting food to a minimum will help you attain your weight goal quickly. As explained above, restrictive eating causes a cascade of hormonal imbalances that can slow weight loss. The recovery solution? Get the carbs right. Yes, despite all the fear around carbohydrate foods, the Femme Fatale often needs them to get her into balance. If you've been restricting carbs for an extended period of time, you may need to add them back in for weight loss, but if you've been eating them for years on end, like the Nurturer, then you'll need to limit them to stimulate fat loss.

Remember, no matter how much weight you lose, or how many bikini sizes you drop, you will never fully reach your crown until you feel totally comfortable in and at ease with your body. As renowned spiritual teacher Marianne Williamson said, "You can't be comfortable in your skin if you think you are your skin." To break this, you will need to practice letting go of the early memories and mind-set that has had a hold on you for so long. When you do this, you'll find that you don't care quite as much if you gain a couple of pounds, and you will exude a natural sense of ease, confidence, and magnetism that makes you feel irresistible.

Step 1: Improve Your Daily Eating Regimen

1. Start each morning with a 4-ounce shot of cucumber juice. Cucumber is rich in potassium and helps to decrease bloating and inflammation so that you can feel more attractive and vitalized. Starting the day with this ritual sets you up for more balanced eating.
2. Do not skip breakfast. Coffee is not breakfast. Fruit is not breakfast. Always eat some form of protein for breakfast, like a plant-based smoothie, a chia seed pudding, or organic eggs.
3. Lunch and dinner should each be composed of seven ingredients: three vegetables, one protein, two fats, one carb. These meals should look like the food plate on page 73.
4. Remember the Rule of 4 when it comes to portion size: a portion equals 4 ounces of protein, ¼ avocado (or other fats), up to 4 cups of vegetables, and ¼ cup of carbs. Yes, you must include those carbs!
5. Don't skip your four p.m. snack. Use this as an opportunity to eat a radiance-boosting snack. A green vegetable juice, some papaya slices with lime, or a crunchy apple is all that you need. If you skip this snack, you'll be hungry before dinner, which increases your risk of mindless or binge eating.
6. In the evening, wind down with a cup of the Femme Fatale's tea.
7. Take the supplements outlined in Step 3 below, which have been designed to improve your mood and decease irritability.

Step 2: Choose the Right Foods

These foods will help to rebalance the Femme Fatale's physical and emotional state, facilitating your ascension to the crown.

1. Eat orange fruits and vegetables daily. This includes carrots, orange bell peppers, peaches, papaya, apricots, citrus, and persimmons. These support the second chakra to decrease judgment and improve your sense of self. Try orange bell peppers in a stir-fry, freshly grated carrot in a nori wrap, or three freshly sliced apricots as an afternoon snack. But don't eat five servings a day! The orange carotenoids, when consumed in excess, can make the skin orange. Remember, it's not "eat this, not that"; it's choosing the right amount.

2. Eat 4 ounces of clean animal protein at lunch and dinner. Don't skimp on the protein. Not only does protein satiate hunger and help the body function, it's also used to create collagen, elastin, and keratin, which keeps your skin supple, bones strong, and hair soft. Eat seafood at least four times a week for its metabolism-boosting properties. You may eat organic tofu and tempeh once a week but not more than that. Eat two eggs up to four times a week. Choose organic poultry when another preferred protein source isn't available.

3. Eat red meat once a week. Femme Fatales with amenorrhea often need to add a weekly serving of red meat to help regulate their menstrual cycle. Grass-fed red meat is not inflammatory. Just pair it with a raw salad loaded with fresh herbs, lemon juice, and a hint of olive oil.

4. Eat ¼ cup of starchy carbs at lunch and dinner. While eating carbs can feel scary for the Femme Fatale, you will always feel more balanced when you add ¼ cup (4 tablespoons) to your meals. Any resistance you feel to eating carbs is pure fear and is holding you back from a peaceful relationship with food. Since you are only dealing with ¼ cup in total, stick with one type of starchy carb per meal—lentils *or* quinoa, not lentils *and* quinoa.

5. Eat beauty-boosting snacks. Think of snacks as an opportunity to add in more nutrients, not something you do out of boredom.

Enjoy fresh raspberries to to bring radiance to the skin or try a turmeric almond milk latte to decrease cellular inflammation.

6. Consider the other archetypes. If your body looks like one of the other archetype's, you can layer on some specifics from their meal guidelines, such as a daily intake of cruciferous vegetables if you tend to carry more fat on your upper thighs, or adding a hint more carbohydrates if you look like the Ethereal and have mood and menstrual irregularities.

Foods that rebalance the Femme Fatale: grilled fish, organic poultry, raw salads, cooked vegetables, fresh herbs, orange fruits and vegetables, nuts, seeds, and a small amount of red meat, grains, legumes, and starchy vegetables.

Foods that should be kept to a minimum: dairy, gluten, soy, and sweets.

FEMME FATALE TEA

This tea is designed to capture the essence of the lovers, muses, and models that inspired the icons of art and literature. Chamomile and lavender are both emotionally harmonizing, while lemongrass decreases exhaustion and bloating. Brahmi, an herb used in many Ayurvedic traditions, helps create higher consciousness to focus on everlasting, etheric beauty. You can find all of the ingredients online. This recipe will make a single 12-ounce serving, but you can mix the tea in bulk and store it in an airtight container.

2 teaspoons *brahmi*
2 teaspoons *dried lemongrass*

1 teaspoon dried chamomile

1 teaspoon dried lavender

Combine the ingredients in a small pot with 12 ounces of hot water. Steep for 5 minutes, then strain into a tea cup. Add more hot water if the tea is too strong.

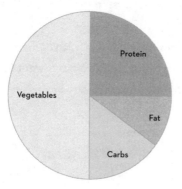

THE FEMME FATALE'S FOOD PLATE

Step 3: Supplement Strategically

The Femme Fatale can support her weight-loss journey by adding in some supportive nutrients:

- **5-HTP:** 5-HTP is the precursor to serotonin, the feel-good neu-rotransmitter. This can help improve the Femme Fatale's mood and reduce her desire for sweet foods and late-night binging. Take 50 mg daily before bed. If you're taking an antidepressant, speak to your physician before using 5-HTP.

- **B Complex:** An activated B complex can help boost the Femme Fatale's energy levels and regulate her hormones. Look for the activated forms such as L-5-MTHF (folate), pyridoxine HCl (B6), and methylcobalamin (B12). Take one after dinner.
- **Magnesium:** Magnesium can help to decrease anxiety. Take 300 mg of magnesium glycinate (or magnesium citrate if constipated) before bed. Magnesium also improves sleep quality.
- **Digestive Enzyme:** Stress can decrease the Femme Fatale's ability to digest her food fully. A digestive enzyme supplement can support her own enzyme production to decrease bloating after meals and enhance the absorption of nutrients. Take this with lunch and dinner.
- **Other Archetypes' Supplements:** If you have a similar body shape to one of the other archetypes, you may want to add in some of their specific supplements until the body has rebalanced itself.

As you ascend toward your crown and abandon the warped eating patterns that have plagued you for years, you can relax some of the meal plan guidelines given above. For instance, you can increase your carbohydrate portion to ½ cup per meal at breakfast, lunch, and dinner. By then you will have come to realize that carbs are not the enemy, and you will trust yourself to consume them in moderation rather than feel you have to maintain an all-or-nothing relationship with them.

EXERCISE SOLUTIONS FOR THE FEMME FATALE

In addition to burning fat and sculpting muscles, the goal of exercise for the Femme Fatale is to help her reconnect with her body through expressive movement. Ideal types of exercise include rebounding, dancing, boxing, swimming, HIIT, plyometrics, bands, and Pilates. Try two dance classes, one intense cardio workout, and one sculpting class per week. On the fifth day, take a yoga class. If using weights, opt for small to medium weights but target a high rep count to help tone and shape your muscles. If you want to build muscle mass, do fewer reps with more weight.

CHAPTER 5

The Ethereal

═══

Juliette is an elite fashion model with a willowy physique, but her stomach is perpetually bloated—especially when she travels frequently for work and doesn't have time to meditate or eat right. Juliette grew up in a Buddhist family eating vegan meals and practicing yoga with her artistic parents. In high school she was considered "weird" so she was relieved that the fashion world accepted her more celestial ways. She knows that New York City is the best home base for her career, but the energy of the city makes her feel like marbles are being thrown at her, and her stomach seems to become even more distended when she is home. She dreams of opening an organic wellness retreat in Costa Rica or Mexico. Juliette is the quintessential Ethereal.

THE ETHEREAL AT HER CROWN:
SPIRITUAL AND SENSITIVE

Ethereals are feminine, whimsical, and enchanting. They're talented, creative, and highly attuned to their surroundings. They possess a refined appreciation of scents, sounds, art, language, and fabric that instinctively pulls them toward artistic and spiritual pursuits. Words like "cosmic," "vibration," and "frequency" are part of their vocabulary. Ethereals are guided through life by their intuition. If something doesn't "feel" right, they won't do it. They can sense the subtle shifts in the unseen. You can't lie to an Ethereal; she will sense it immediately. She may even appear to have psychic abilities.

Ethereals have historically been thought of as eccentric, woo-woo, and "out there," but as society is starting to appreciate the power of intuition, Ethereals are now considered the "cool" girls. The fashion and wellness industries have positioned Ethereals as the girls to emulate with their free-spirited ways. As alluring as the aspirational images of boho beauties lounging in a riad in Marrakech are—particularly for a stressed-out Wonder Woman—the essence of the Ethereal is not about what she wears or how she speaks. It's about the expression of herself through her intuition and a connection with a higher realm. Ethereals unequivocally believe that there is something intangible guiding and supporting them.

Ethereals see underlying harmony as the structure of the universe. They don't understand why people argue, fight, and engage in conflict. They look at every human, plant, and animal as connected; when one suffers, everyone does. This makes them very sensitive. But if they do not understand their sensitivity, they can absorb other people's emotions and become teary for no apparent reason. An Ethereal at her crown has learned to distinguish which emotions are hers and warrant inward investigation, and which emotions are from an external source and can be released. When she is not at her crown, she struggles to discern the difference, and every upsetting emotion can feel like a weight pinning her to the floor.

The Ethereal feels constrained by excess structure and logic. Taking a nine-to-five job is death to her soul, even if it takes her out of financial straits. She fears that it will corrupt her creative expression, which, for her, is worse than being monetarily poor. But when the creative chemistry of an Ethereal is allowed to flourish, particularly in the corporate world, it can be transformative for her and the people and institutions around her. Ethereals make life rich and colorful, and without them, life is black and white, rigid and contained.

Ethereals rarely hold resentments or grudges. They are forgiving and generous to others. This is one of the reasons for their low body weight and wraithlike quality—there's less emotional baggage holding them down. When an Ethereal is at her crown, she is guided by her intuition and knows how to balance the demands of her outer world with the needs of her most spiritual self. She is soulful and successful and appears to float through life with an ethereal tranquility.

Ethereals on Earth include Fiona Apple, Kate Moss, Joan Didion, Edie Sedgwick, Carrie Bradshaw, Holly Golightly, and your artistic girlfriend who is traveling the world in a free-spirited way.

THE BELIEF SYSTEM:
"MY INTUITION IS MY GIFT"

Ethereals believe their intuition is always right, but the *interpretation* of their intuition may not be. It may simply be a thought emerging from their subconscious, which is filtered by their experiences, particularly their childhood wounds. These wayward "intuitions" can make them feel scattered, spacey, overwhelmed, and unsure of what direction to take.

When the Ethereal's intuition isn't grounded with intellect, financial success can allude her. She can swing from one idea to the next depending on what she "hears" from her intuition, never sticking with one thing long enough to achieve stability. As she believes her intuition is always right, she can fall into the trap of not considering the financial feasibility of each project. My client Sadie, a designer of yoga wear, wanted to be a sound healer, develop meditation retreats, create jewelry, design scents, and bring women together for goddess tribes. While these ideas complemented her clothing line, and were all possible, Sadie struggled to keep her business afloat, let alone have the capacity or money to follow through on these other ideas. With so many goals she was stuck in inertia, not knowing what direction to take. Just as Wonder Woman overvalues her intellect, the Ethereal can overvalue her intuition. Both are guidance tools and they need each other to be effective. Sadie needed to consider the practical aspects of what her inner self was telling her to do.

On the other hand, if an Ethereal does not fully recognize her intuitive gift as her power source, she can unwittingly subjugate it to "fit in" to a world that values logic, looks, and finances over spiritual pursuits. My client Nina pursued a career as a corporate lawyer because that's what was expected of a good Jewish girl from New York. But she is also a gifted poet and writer, and her career choice neutralized her Ethereal ways and exponentially increased her anxiety. She was left wondering, "Am I good at anything?"

An Ethereal can find herself obsessed with her body and food, exhibiting Femme Fatale traits, not realizing that she's abandoned her intuitive essence. Not being able to exercise her true nature, she feels trapped and forlorn, and her self-esteem and self-worth become fragile and tender. Her physical body soon follows suit.

THE ETHEREAL ARCHETYPE: SIXTH, SEVENTH, AND EIGHTH CHAKRAS

The Ethereal is guided by the super-consciousness—the sixth, seventh, and eighth chakras, which represent intuition, insight, and connection to a purpose beyond the visible. The sixth chakra is located at the third eye, which is the point between the two eyebrows and is associated with the pituitary gland. The seventh chakra is located at the crown of your head and is associated with the pineal gland.

The eighth chakra is your aura. The purity of the super-consciousness is only accessed when the lower chakras are balanced. When the Ethereal falls into self-doubt and emotional instability, she needs to reconnect with the sixth, seventh, and eighth chakras and not float away into the celestial sphere. All archetypes can access these chakras, but the Ethereal is more attuned to them.

The super-consciousness is represented by the colors indigo, purple, and white. When the Ethereal needs to balance her intuition with her rational, more cognitive side, she can eat more purple and white plant foods. Most of us know that blueberries can improve our brain power, and that's exactly how the Ethereal can use them. Purple cabbage, plums, purple grapes, leeks, onions, and potatoes (purple and white) can be used to enhance her cognition and rational thought. When she is lacking inspiration, she can use these same foods to strengthen her insight and wisdom. Wearing white enhances her radiance, while wearing purple helps to fine-tune her consciousness.

CHILDHOOD PATTERNS: FROM INTROSPECTIVE TO INTUITIVE TO "AM I CRAZY?"

Ethereal girls are inquisitive and embody innocent curiosity. They're often introspective and try to process what they see and feel in the world. They may have been considered eccentric and learned to retreat into their inner thoughts. As painful as this might have been, it has shaped the Ethereal into the highly attuned woman she is today. Now she can sense things before they happen.

If the Ethereal's parents nurtured her dreamy and imaginative ways, she will be bolder and more grounded than her Ethereal sisters who have learned to hide their intuitive gifts. In some extreme cases, Ethereal children can be put on a stimulant like Ritalin to force them to concentrate and focus. This is like shoving a square peg into a round hole; the stimulant will stunt her creative development in favor of concentration. How this ultimately affects the Ethereal as an adult is unknown, yet I suspect her repressed creativity will lead to the symptoms of withdrawal, sadness, skin breakouts, and digestive issues I see with Ethereal women who've disowned their intuitive ways.

If the Ethereal didn't feel supported as a child, she may have layered on the Wonder Woman's traits of perfection and found herself desperately seeking attention and approval by over-performing. When my client Susan, a dancer, was a child, she was constantly in motion—jumping, dancing, stretching, playing, and expressing herself through her body. Her parents didn't know how to respond to this outpouring of creative energy and encouraged her to develop other skills and to stay still. Susan did as she was told, but because her primary mode of expression had been shut down, she shut down, too. She had learned through her parents' messaging that moving around freely was "wrong" and that staying still and being perfect was "right." This made her feel like she wasn't normal and that her parents would not love her unless she abandoned who she was. She felt unaccepted and unworthy and tried to literally disappear by adopting disordered eating behaviors and exercising obsessively. It was only when we worked out together that she saw this pattern and was able to discard her need for perfection and lean into the rhythm of life. Her dance performances also improved because she trusted that her unique expression of the dance was what was captivating, not the perfection of the moves.

OUT OF BALANCE: "I FEEL ANXIOUS, SPACEY, AND SENSITIVE"

Like the other archetypes, an out-of-balance Ethereal will either operate in the amplification, always believing her intuition, whether it is right or not, or in the withdrawal, ignoring her instincts in favor of a more intellectual and rational outlook.

In the amplification, she's on a quest to obey her intuition and avoid anything that may turn it off. She disconnects from reality, feels ungrounded, and becomes easily distracted. Depression, vertigo, inability to concentrate, skin breakouts, and irritable bowel syndrome (IBS) are common symptoms. There are so many discombobulated thoughts running through her mind, she can't make sense of it all, and she can struggle to make decisions. She may also shun the world, terrified that if she joins the mainstream her extrasensory abilities will be switched off. She can go to great lengths to avoid this integration, including secluding herself in ashrams, meditating for hours on end, and forgetting to eat. One of my Ethereal clients used the quote from French philosopher Pierre Teilhard de Chardin, "We are spiritual beings having a human experience," to justify her disconnection from the human world. *But, I'm really a spirit!* While she is a spirit, she is *also* a human being and therefore needs to remind herself to do human things like sleep, eat, foster meaningful relationships, and offer compassion to a fractured world. For the Ethereal to flourish, she needs to be centered, grounded, and present. Embodying the positive attributes of the other archetypes can help her achieve this.

In the withdrawal, the Ethereal has switched off her intuition in an attempt to be accepted by a world that has historically valued intellect and physical appearance over the mystical. She may struggle with anxiety, sadness, and digestive issues from compressed creative expression, as Nina the corporate lawyer and Susan the dancer did. The solution for her is to recognize that, like the bird in a gilded cage, her wings have been clipped. Once she understands that her instinctive way is to be expansive, dreamy, and imaginative, she'll be like the ugly duckling realizing she's a swan. She opens up, her creative fire is stoked, and she reclaims her dreamy, celestial ways. It's magnificent.

When my client Laura realized she was an Ethereal operating in Wonder Woman mode, she had an epiphany. She no longer needed to own a big company to feel successful. Instead, she dropped the clients who were causing her to reach for the booze every night. She reconnected with her love of surfing and hiking and lived a life unburdened by unnecessary demands and rules. Her anxiety, exhaustion, and muffin top all disappeared.

EATING BEHAVIOR: "I'M SO SENSITIVE TO FOOD!"

The Ethereal is highly sensitive to the vibration of food, and eating the standard American diet is even more deleterious for her than to the other archetypes. Even though a junky diet will leave anyone feeling bloated, depressed, and fatigued, the Ethereal will feel these effects first. An Ethereal can also have multiple allergies and food sensitivities because of her more finely tuned frequency. Her physical body rejects chemicals and sends her into a hyperactive tailspin.

When my Ethereal friend was working for a woman's beauty magazine (which is naturally out of alignment for an Ethereal because the focus on physical beauty is foreign to her), she'd eat junky food to escape the disappointment of the career she had chosen. It was only when she was courageous enough to leave her job for more creative endeavors that her food choices changed and she understood that she had turned to these unhealthy foods to feel numb.

If you are an Ethereal and are absorbed in what you're creating, you may forget to eat. This can trigger blood-sugar imbalances and anxiety. It's vital that you eat clean, healthy food every few hours to keep yourself connected to the physical plane.

THE CHALLENGE FOR THE ETHEREAL: TO INTEGRATE THE INTUITIVE WITH THE INTELLECTUAL

My friend Shiva Rose is an Ethereal at her crown. She describes the metamorphosis that occurred when she was going through a divorce and raising two children. She couldn't just drift away into the mystical world. She had responsibilities. She needed to create a home, make money, and be a mother. She learned to get back to the earth. She purchased a place in Los Angeles where she could raise chickens, plant a vegetable and herb garden, and bask in the Californian sunshine. She also created a high-end organic skin-care line with roses sourced from Italy. She describes this as balance and choice. She can be ethereal and float out into the astral world with intense breath work or she can be grounded by gardening and cooking with spices and herbs. Grounding has expanded her life, not compressed it.

Similarly, when Sadie harnessed her inner Wonder Woman by integrating intellect with her intuition, she was able to apply financial logic to her creative ideas and rapidly increase the profitability of her yoga apparel business. Today she has a flourishing business that has expanded to include all of the things she wanted to develop.

The first mini-challenge for the Ethereal is to plan a day of activities and to follow through on all of them. Although you may feel some resistance toward this since you prefer to follow your whims, this exercise will help you become more structured and show you that you won't die from boredom if you stick to a plan. You can choose any activities you want, but you must write them down, then follow the schedule precisely. Doing this one day a week for four weeks will help activate your inner Wonder Woman.

To ascend to your crown, you must believe that applying logic to your creative ideas won't distort them. Rather, it helps discern which are valid and which are not. When you simultaneously blend your intuition with your intellect, there's nothing you can't bring to fruition. To help you get there, you can activate the positive attributes of the other archetypes:

- Layer in the earthiness of the Nurturer by planting herbs and flowers and sourcing your food from a local farmers' market.
- Embody the Wonder Woman's resilience and become stronger and more robust in your thinking.
- Embrace the body awareness of the balanced Femme Fatale so you don't forget that you are also a physical being.

When you layer in these attributes, you become a source of feminine inspiration. You become the mystical muse for your archetype sisters.

THE ETHEREAL FOOD PRESCRIPTION

The Ethereal is naturally lean, with a willowy and light physique supported by long, slender muscles. Your physiology is naturally balanced and can process food more efficiently thanks to well-regulated insulin levels and thyroid function. If you do gain weight, it is usually the result of relying on starchy and sugary foods in an effort to numb your sensitivity to the energies and emotions of others.

Even so, I have never met an Ethereal with the body shape of a Nurturer. My friend Madeline is able to connect with the angels, but this doesn't make her an Ethereal. She's a gifted healer who imparts unconditional love and has a sturdier body. She is a Nurturer who has ascended closer to her crown and is therefore able to tap into her innate spiritual energy. If you identify psychologically as an Ethereal but your body looks more like that of a Nurturer or Wonder Woman, you are probably not an Ethereal and should not follow her meal plan, which is the least restrictive and therefore less suitable if you are trying to lose weight. Instead, follow the meal plans for the archetype who best matches your body shape.

It's not entirely clear why Ethereals are blessed with a body that burns fat easily, but my guess is that it's because they are more in tune with their energetic body, which helps balance the physical body. Our energetic body is invisible and connected to the spiritual world, so other archetypes are prone to neglect it because they can't see it. Ethereals, however, are more aware of their energy and, when they sense an imbalance, can work to correct it through practices like meditation, yoga, and breath work. All of the archetypes can benefit from this type of spiritual work, and in Part III, I will discuss why integrating them into your life will ultimately put you on a path to achieving weight loss and a better sense of overall health and well-being.

IMBALANCES: ESTROGEN, AND THE GUT MICROBIOME

Due to your low body weight, you can have hormonal issues caused by low levels of estrogen. Too little estrogen can lead to a variety of symptoms such as amenorrhea, depression, dry skin, insomnia, low libido, and infertility. Increasing your carbohydrate intake can help boost the amount of free estrogen in your body.

Ethereals also regularly suffer from constipation and bloating, often caused by an out-of-balance gut microbiome that is riddled with pathogenic bacteria and yeast. These microbes are usually beneficial and, when in balance, the gut microbiome helps with a variety of important bodily functions, including stabilizing mood, controlling hunger, stimulating fat burning, supporting the thyroid, and regulating sex hormone levels. But, thanks in no small part to the rapid industrialization of our food system, which introduced antibiotics into the standard American diet, many of these good bacteria have been killed off or mutated into pathogenic yeast, bacteria, or parasites that wreak havoc on your body, especially your digestion. Excess refined carbohydrates can disrupt the delicate balance of good bacteria to bad bacteria. When you feel spacey or depressed, you can make poor dietary choices, which further upset the gut microbiome.

While Ethereals are typically lean, a disrupted gut microbiome has been found to play a role in weight gain. The link between the gut microbiome and weight gain became unassailable in 2004, when researchers took the gut microbiota from regular mice and inserted it into germ-free mice. The germ-free mice had a 60 percent increase in body fat and insulin resistance within just two weeks![1] The researchers concluded that the gut bacteria played an instrumental role in how we store body fat. The researchers then took the microbiota from both the lean mice and obese mice and inoculated the germ-free mice. The result: the microbiota from the obese mice caused greater weight gain despite the mice eating less food and exercising more![2]

If you are an Ethereal who is prone to constipation, bloating, flatulence, or other digestive issues, chances are, your gut microbiome is to blame. Pathogenic yeast is most often the cause, and I recommend taking specific supplements to kill off the mutated forms of yeast. Bad bacteria and parasites may also be contributing to your symptoms, and if your symptoms don't resolve after the anti-yeast protocol discussed in the supplement section, I suggest you work with a functional medicine practitioner or naturopath who can test your gut microbial composition.

THE ETHEREAL'S MEAL PLAN

Because Ethereals are better able to regulate their body weight—and may even have trouble keeping weight on—you are able to eat more healthy carbs than the other archetypes. Increasing the amount of starchy vegetables, legumes, and grains in your diet will increase your estrogen levels, which may help alleviate some of your other symptoms. Carbs also help the Ethereal feel grounded. Since you may be prone to feeling scattered—especially when out of balance—these foods help to keep you connected to the earth.

The guidelines below outline the general principles around which you should structure your meals. A ten-day plan, which incorporates these concepts, is on page 162.

Step 1: Improve Your Daily Eating Regimen

1. Start each morning with a 4-ounce shot of aloe vera juice to help support your digestive system.
2. Ethereals are the only archetype who can start the day with a serving of good-quality carbs like warm quinoa with cinnamon and coconut milk or organic eggs on gluten-free toast. An Ethereal who eats only fruit for breakfast will find herself feeling more scattered later in the day.
3. Eat seven ingredients at lunch and dinner: three vegetables, one protein, two fats, and ¾ cup of carbohydrates. These meals should look like the food plate on page 90.
4. Don't forget to eat. Make time for your three meals and two snacks each day; otherwise your body will not get the nutrients it needs to function properly.
5. Wind down your evenings with a cup of tea designed for the Ethereal.
6. Take the supplements outlined in Step 3 below to restore and repair your gut microbiome.

Step 2: Choose the Right Foods

Specific foods can help to rebalance the Ethereal's physical and energetic state. The suggestions below augment the general recommendations made in Part II to address the Ethereal's particular concerns.

1. Eat cooked vegetables. Ethereals tend to gravitate toward more of a raw diet, but cooked vegetables are more grounding and easier on the digestive system. If you are deciding between a raw salad and wok-tossed vegetables, then the latter is a better choice. This doesn't mean that the only vegetables you eat have to be cooked, but do include them in the diet. Root vegetables are particularly beneficial for the Ethereal because they keep you rooted to the earth.

2. Eat one white or purple fruit or vegetable daily. These colors are associated with the six, seventh, and eighth chakras, so incorporating these foods into your diet will help bring clarity to your intuition.

3. Add your carbs. If you are the rare Ethereal who is trying to lose weight, start by eating ½ cup of carbs at lunch and at dinner. This is twice the recommended serving for the other archetypes, but it is necessary for you to feel centered. You can also eat carbs for breakfast, like gluten-free granola, once a week. If you are eating for maintenance, you can up your intake to ¾ cup at breakfast and 1½ cups at lunch and dinner. You can eat two types of carbohydrates at meals, too. Think dahl with roasted yams, sprouted brown rice with black beans, or gluten-free tartine with hummus.

4. Eat red meat up to three times a week. Red meat is very grounding and helps with muscle development for the Ethereal. Try grass-fed steak, a lamb ragu over butternut squash noodles, and grass-fed bison tacos with sauerkraut.

5. Soy and dairy can be consumed, provided it is organic. Organic soy can help increase your usually low estrogen levels, so you can eat tofu and tempeh up to three times a week, if you desire. I recommend that all archetypes go on a dairy hiatus for four weeks, but after this period, you are the only archetype that can consume good-quality dairy on a regular basis because you are the least sensitive to dairy's insulin response. High-quality, organic dairy products can be consumed up to three times a week.

6. Snack on nuts. Nuts are a great way for the Ethereal to feel grounded. You can have them twice a day—once as a snack and once in a meal.

7. Eat fermented foods at least once a week. Foods like sauerkraut, kimchi, miso soup, unpasteurized olives and pickles, kombucha, and kefir contain live bacteria that help replete a damaged microbiome. Add sauerkraut to organic eggs, have miso soup as a snack, or add kefir to your morning smoothie.

In summary, the Ethereal's meal plan is the most abundant. Your focus should be on eating regularly and favoring foods that help you feel rooted to the earth such as cooked vegetables, red meat, legumes, grains, starchy vegetables, and nuts. If your microbiome has been damaged, fermented foods can also help you replenish the good microbes in the gut.

Foods to limit: Sweets

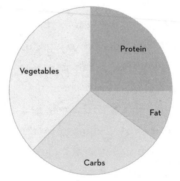

THE ETHEREAL'S FOOD PLATE

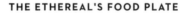

THE ETHEREAL'S TEA

The Ethereal's tea is inspired by the Jazz Age in Paris when Zelda Fitzgerald was marginalized for her uninhibited and iridescent ways. This tea will leave you wild while providing enough earthiness to keep you sane. The lemongrass and ginger are energizing, while the burdock root supports liver rejuvenation and the absorption of nutrients. Orange peel helps fat digestion to improve skin clarity. These can be enjoyed any time of day, but this tea is especially good to drink in the evening to help re-center you at the end of the day. This recipe makes a single 12-ounce serving, but you can increase the quantities of the ingredients and store them in an airtight container for later use. All ingredients can be found online.

2 teaspoons burdock root
One 1-inch piece fresh ginger, chopped
1 teaspoon dried lemongrass
1 teaspoon orange peel

Combine the ingredients in a small pot with 12 ounces of hot water. Steep for 5 minutes, then strain into a tea cup. Add more hot water if the tea is too strong.

Step 3: Supplement Strategically

The Ethereal's supplements are designed to decrease bloating, increase energy levels, and improve your mood.

- **Candida Control:** This is a specific supplement by Enzyme Science that is designed to kill off pathogenic yeast in the gut microbiome that may be contributing to your bloating. Take this for six weeks and follow the instructions on the bottle.
- **Probiotic:** Repopulate the gut microbiome with a twelve-strain probiotic. Look for at least 25 billion CFUs (colony-forming units) or find a fermented probiotic like Dr. Ohhira to help stimulate the growth of bacteria. Take daily.

- **B Complex:** Take an activated B complex to help boost energy levels and regulate hormone levels. Look for the activated forms such as L-5-MTHF (folate), pyridoxine HCl (B6), and methylcobalamin (B12). Take one after dinner.
- **Magnesium Citrate:** Magnesium citrate helps stimulate peristalsis to promote regular bowel movements and decrease constipation. Magnesium also encourages a deeper level of sleep. Take 300 mg before bed.
- **5-HTP:** 5-HTP is the precursor to serotonin and if you are feeling blue or anxious, or can't sleep, experiment with 50 mg before bed. If you are taking an antidepressant, check with your physician before taking 5-HTP.

When the Ethereal is in balance, you are at one with your strong spiritual side but have your feet firmly planted on the ground. You prioritize nourishing your body as much as you do your creativity and soul and have increased energy and attention that you can devote to your many pursuits. Your belly is free of bloat and your mood is balanced and calm.

EXERCISE SOLUTIONS FOR THE ETHEREAL

Since the Ethereal rarely needs to burn body fat, intense cardio classes aren't necessary for her. If you're an Ethereal, try TRX classes, barre classes, and Pilates classes, which will help reshape your naturally thin muscles. Use small weights and target a high rep count, and take any combination of these five times a week. You can also use exercise as an opportunity to connect with nature. Hike, surf, swim in the ocean, or take an outdoor tennis or yoga class. Opt for these on the days when you're not taking other classes.

PART II

FEED

YOUR BODY

WITHOUT

FEAR

Now that you know the formula for how to eat for your archetype, you need to know the details about how to incorporate various types of food into your diet and why. What specific foods should you eat and which should you avoid? What types of proteins, fats, and carbs should you favor, and why are they necessary for a balanced diet? Does when and how frequently you eat matter? What about treat foods? How can you enjoy them while still losing weight? The goal of this section is to arm you with the information you need to make better decisions about your meals without stressing or feeling like you constantly need to deprive yourself if you want to lose weight.

I also want to bust some of the most damaging myths about what makes a food "good" or "bad" so you can let go of your food fears and develop healthier, more sustainable eating behaviors. I've designed the Archetype Model to include as many different types of foods as possible. Too many popular programs these days eliminate foods that are good for you because there is a very small possibility they may exacerbate symptoms in people who are unwell. For instance, people with rheumatoid arthritis are often told to avoid tomatoes because they may heighten their inflammatory symptoms. This does not mean that tomatoes are inflammatory (in fact, they are not), but rather, in this particular disease, they may not be as beneficial as an alternative vegetable. For people who are healthy, tomatoes are a very enjoyable way to take in the phytonutrient lycopene. And who doesn't love a fresh heirloom tomato salad with olive oil and sea salt?

Overly restrictive diets not only deny us beneficial nutrients, they also create an unnecessary fear around food. If you already struggle with negative feelings about your self-worth, you don't need any additional anxiety when you sit down at the dinner table. You need a meal plan that fits around your life and gives you everything you need to be beautiful and brainy. While you may stick to a crash or elimination diet long enough to shed a few pounds, you'll never maintain this program over the long haul; it's just too limited. The Archetype Model is meant to be a lifestyle, and if you're going to stick to a plan for the long haul, you need to feel like you're not missing out or depriving yourself. You need to develop a peaceful, lasting relationship with food.

While each of the archetype-specific meal plans has been customized to address the issues most common to each archetype, they are all based on certain foundational truths and principles about how the body processes different foods. Understanding the role these foods play in our health will allow you to let go of any fears or misconceptions you may have been harboring that have caused you to see food as a source of anxiety instead of what it actually is: a form of nourishment that helps you achieve wellness.

CHAPTER 6

Food Fundamentals

═══

While each archetype has a slightly different set of nutritional requirements, certain foundational food principles apply to everyone. Think of these principles as the foundation of the house, and the archetype-specific guidelines as the decor that reflects your personality. They are both essential for eating in a way that is supportive to your unique biochemistry. Some of the principles I include in this chapter will sound familiar—you already know you need to eat your vegetables—while others will be more surprising. All of these Food Fundamentals are easy to implement and serve as the base for eating for life. If at any time your archetype-specific guidelines feel overwhelming, just return to this chapter. This is a lifestyle diet, not a short-term fix or detox.

Both the Food Fundamentals and the archetype-specific meal plans are designed to incorporate as many different foods as possible. Your body is very smart and, because it needs a wide array of nutrients for optimal health, it will produce dopamine, the pleasure neurotransmitter, when you eat new foods. The only other way you produce dopamine from food is by eating sugar. So if you don't want to submit to sugar cravings, eat a wide variety of foods! That being said, when I say "food," I don't simply mean "something that is edible." Your diet needs to consist of real, whole foods—things that exist in nature—not the processed or packaged kind. Not only should you be eating real fruits, vegetables, fats, proteins, and carbs, but you should strive to consume the highest quality you can find. Opt for organic, sustainable, and/or grass-fed when given the choice. If that's not possible, don't sweat it. Just stick to the Food Fundamentals as best as you can.

THE FOOD FUNDAMENTALS

Only Eat Food You'd Photograph

This does not mean you need to Instagram every meal you eat (though if you want to, tag me!), but it does serve as a useful guideline by which to measure the purity of your food. When our meals are rich in bright colors and textures, we're more attracted to them—and with good reason. The denser the color of a fruit or vegetable, the more phytonutrients (beneficial plant molecules) it contains. A green salad interspersed with yellow beets, red onion, and purple potatoes is more appealing to the eye than a white potato salad with mayo and celery. It also contains a greater array of phytonutrients, all supporting the body in a unique way. And you've probably noticed the difference in color between wild-caught salmon and the farm-raised variety. The wild-caught salmon contains the antioxidant astaxanthin, which protects your cells from free-radical damage and helps improve your skin's elasticity and moisture levels. The farmed salmon doesn't contain this antioxidant and thus has fewer beneficial beauty properties.

If you eat depleted food, that's how you'll feel, physically and mentally. When you eat pretty food, you'll *feel* pretty. Similarly, if you want to be happy, eat food that has been made with joy—food made with love feels very different from a prepackaged frozen meal. In essence, match the energetics of the food to how you want to look and feel.

Fast for Twelve Hours a Day

Don't panic—you will be sleeping for most of this fasting period! I want you to keep your meals to a twelve-hour period and fast for the other twelve hours of the day. That means if you eat dinner at eight p.m., you'll eat breakfast at eight a.m. If you eat dinner at six p.m., you'll eat breakfast at six a.m. When you fast for twelve hours between dinner and breakfast, your body's metabolic processes are optimized, inflammation is reduced, and fat loss is enhanced. In a recent study, scientists found that mice who fasted for twelve to fifteen hours a day were thinner and healthier than those that were able to eat at all hours, even when they consumed the same number of calories.[1]

Do not, however, fast for sixteen hours (and restrict your eating to an eight-hour window) by skipping breakfast the next morning. This is a technique that some people use to control weight loss, but this strategy will ultimately backfire by interfering with the body's ability to regulate its glucose levels. When you skip meals, your adrenal glands will respond by putting sugar into the blood even though you didn't eat. That's because you need to maintain a minimum level of glucose in the blood or you will become hypoglycemic. Your adrenal glands control your stress response, and skipping a meal depletes your supply of stress hormones, meaning you'll have less stress hormones available to help you cope with the ups and downs of the day. Twelve on/twelve off is a reasonable schedule that feels easy to follow. Just make sure to finish your last meal or snack at least two hours before you go to sleep so that your body is not trying to do two incongruent processes—digesting food and sleeping—at the same time.

Eat Five Times a Day

To keep hunger at bay, I want you to eat three meals and two snacks—no more, no less—during the twelve hours of the day when you consume your meals. Do not graze; you'll lose track of how much you eat. Eating

scheduled meals and snacks will make it easier to monitor your food intake, and it will also help stave off cravings since you'll be eating regularly. Work backward from the time you go to sleep to figure out what eating intervals work best for you. For instance, your meals might be laid out as follows:

EARLY RISER

6:00 A.M.	7:00 A.M.	10:00 A.M.	1:00 P.M.	4:00 P.M.	7:00 P.M.	10:00 P.M.
Wake up	Breakfast	Snack	Lunch	Snack	Dinner	Bed

NIGHT OWL

8:00 A.M.	10:00 A.M.	1:00 P.M.	4:00 P.M.	8:00 P.M.	10:00 P.M.	12:00 A.M.
Wake up	Breakfast	Lunch	Snack	Dinner	Snack	Bed

If you're not hungry for a snack, either your meals are too large or you've trained your body not to get hungry, which is not necessarily a good thing. If you're not used to eating a snack, I urge you to try it. Snacks give you the opportunity to take in more nutrients, provided you are following Food Fundamental "When Snacking, Calories Matter."

Breakfast Is the Least Important Meal of the Day

Contrary to popular opinion, breakfast is *not* the most important meal of the day. (That is a myth created to get you to eat packaged cereal!) Your appetite-suppressing hormones, GLP-1 and CCK, are highest during the

early part of the day, which is why you often don't feel hungry when you first wake up even though you haven't eaten for twelve hours. It also explains why you can eat a light breakfast and still feel satiated. Light, however, doesn't mean you should only eat fruit. Fruit is metabolized within sixty minutes and will leave you feeling hungrier than before you ate. (Fruit is fine as a snack later in the day when you just need something to hold you over from lunch to dinner, but not as the base for starting your day.)

If you want to speed up the body's ability to burn fat, eat a protein-based breakfast, like organic eggs, a plant-based protein smoothie, or chia seed pudding. Protein activates the hormone glucagon, which helps to burn body fat. Eating protein for breakfast has also been shown to decrease the number of calories you consume throughout the rest of the day. In a 1999 study at Harvard University, participants were fed breakfasts of instant oatmeal, steel-cut oatmeal, or a vegetable omelet with a side of fruit and were then allowed to consume all the food they wanted for the rest of the day. Even though each breakfast had the same number of calories, when the participants ate the instant oatmeal, they devoured a whopping 500 to 600 more calories throughout the day than on the days that they ate the omelet. When the same subjects ate the steel-cut oats, they consumed an additional 300 calories compared to the day they ate eggs and fruit.[2] This increased hunger is one of the main reasons why I don't suggest eating oats (instant or steel cut) for breakfast, no matter how "healthy" you've heard they are. What's more, a fasting body is particularly sensitive to sugar and carbs, so if you eat only oats, cereal, toast, or pancakes for breakfast, you'll tip your body in favor of fat storage, not fat burning.

I recommend eating light to heavy, with your lightest meal at breakfast and largest meal at dinner. Most people are hungrier and more relaxed in the evening than they are in the morning, and the body secretes more digestive enzymes when it is in a relaxed state. These enzymes help break down food into its individual components so that the nutrients can be better absorbed and utilized by the body. Just don't eat a massive meal right before bed! See Food Fundamental "Fast for Twelve Hours a Day."

Eat Your Veggies!

You already know you should eat your vegetables, but I want to get specific here:

1. Eat at least half a plate—about 2 to 4 cups—of vegetables at both lunch and dinner.
2. Include three different vegetables at each of these meals. Only by eating three different vegetables will you get the diversity of phytonutrients needed to optimize your vitality, mind, and health.

Eating this way isn't complicated, but it does require you to pay attention to your food, especially when ordering out. Too often, for instance, a menu will list something as a "salad" that only contains one vegetable. A kale salad with walnuts, dried cranberries, and feta cheese is not a salad; it's a cheese plate served on a bed of kale! A kale salad with red onion and yellow peppers, or even a steak accompanied by a side of mixed vegetables, would be a better choice.

Eating three vegetables does not mean you can only eat salad. You could have a vegetable soup made with organic carrots, leeks, and celery or a veggie plate made with ruby-red heirloom tomatoes, French radish, and grilled asparagus.

Portion Size Matters

I don't want you to count calories at meals, as doing so distorts how you view food. I want you to focus on the composition of the meal, not numbers. But that doesn't mean you can just eat unlimited quantities of healthy foods and lose weight. To lose weight, you must also consider the *amount* of food you eat. Your hands serve as a proxy for gauging caloric intake without counting calories. Simply hold your hands out side by side, palms up. This represents the area your meal should cover. The left hand is the portion size for vegetables and it can be overflowing. The right hand is for all of the other ingredients that comprise your meal—carbs, protein, and fat—and the precise balance of those elements will depend on your archetype. I once had twins in my office, and one of them was twenty pounds heavier than the other. Not surprisingly, her hands were larger than her sister's, confirming that she needed more food to support her slightly larger frame.

When Snacking, Calories Matter

While I just said you don't have to count calories at meals, I *do* want you to consider them when choosing your snacks. It's very easy to go overboard on snacks, and that can be the difference between weight loss and weight gain. For each of your two daily snacks, the number of calories should be no greater than the equivalent of your *goal* weight in pounds. If you want to get to 120 pounds, eat two 120-calorie snacks. If your goal is 150 pounds, eat two 150-calorie snacks. When snacking, opt for fruits, fats, or vegetables, not protein or carbs. Unless you're training intensely or are looking to build muscle mass, you don't need more protein than what you are getting from your meals, so no snacks of turkey jerky, hard-boiled eggs, or chicken slices. Likewise, limit carbs to mealtimes, as carbs are the levers for weight loss and weight gain—in general, the more you eat, the harder it is to lose. Instead, try half an avocado with lime, maca-dusted hazelnuts (fourteen is about 120 calories), 2 tablespoons of turmeric-spiced pumpkin seeds, 12 ounces of green vegetable juice or bone broth, a matcha latte made with creamy cashew milk, four fresh figs, a pear with tahini, or a small chia seed pudding with fresh apricots.

Say No to Gluten and Dairy (Temporarily)

I know I mentioned earlier that I wouldn't restrict the foods you can eat, but I have found that temporarily removing gluten and dairy from your diet can help rebalance the body and make it easier to lose weight. Once you've improved your body's resilience, you will be able to tolerate a greater diversity of foods, including high-quality forms of gluten and dairy. To do this, however, the body may require a small break to correct itself since these foods can trigger inflammation and interfere with cellular processes that govern your physical body and emotional state.

If you're unhappy with how you look and feel, experiment with a four-week gluten and dairy hiatus, particularly if you haven't tried this before. Just take out the obvious—no pasta, bread, cakes, cookies, milk, yogurt, cheese, or ice cream—and see what happens. If your brain fogginess, cravings, fatigue, and bloating dissipate during this time, I highly recommend you stay gluten- and dairy-free for at least another eight months. This is typically enough time to down-regulate the body's overactive immune response to these foods. After that, you can gradually reintroduce gluten and dairy as long as they are organic so that you are not consuming pesticides and growth hormones. All of the archetype meal plans are gluten- and dairy-free to help get you started.

Don't Eat to Cheat

Although your archetype meal plans are meant to be followed for life, I do not want you to feel like you need to "cheat" in order to enjoy foods that fall outside of these recommendations. That's why I strongly encourage you to enjoy one pleasure meal each week. This is not a "cheat" meal; it's part of your archetype's plan and is meant to be savored and enjoyed without guilt.

There are no rules about what to eat for your pleasure meals but Chapter 12, "Permission for Pleasure," provides suggestions on how to structure them. I've had a number of clients who worry that opening the door to treats, however infrequently, will derail their diets, but I promise this is not the case. The archetype plan is designed to help you adopt better eating habits that you can sustain for the long term. At the same time, these meals will stop your body from calibrating to what you're eating by adding variety into your diet, top up your glycogen (stored energy) levels, and help you avoid that much-feared weight-loss plateau.

The goal of these plans is to help you form a peaceful relationship with food, which means not being afraid of it. I don't ever want you to feel guilty because you ate something you weren't "supposed" to eat. If the idea of a treat meal has you panicking because you worry it will set off a binge, trust yourself more. Turn to the exercises in Part III on healing the mind to help you if you need support.

Get in the Kitchen

Thankfully, we've come a long way from the time when women were expected to make all of their family's meals, but that doesn't mean we should give up cooking altogether. You already know that homemade meals are better for you than frozen, processed meals or takeout, but there are other benefits to cooking as well. When you smell food cooking, your digestive juices start to secrete. This primes your body for enhanced digestion, including better nutrient absorption. If you get a bloated belly after eating, this is one way to decrease the likelihood of that happening. Slow down, savor the aromas, and relish the knowledge that when you eat a meal you've prepared from real ingredients, you're taking in more minerals, vitamins, phytonutrients, and amino acids to support your biochemistry.

If gourmet cooking is not part of your skill set, don't worry; none of the meals I suggest require more than a few minutes of prep and a handful of ingredients. Foods picked from the earth and grown without pesticides and chemicals require very little dressing up; a splash of olive oil, lemon juice, and sea salt is all that is often needed.

The Food Fundamentals are principles to live by, not commandments etched in stone. If you're not able to eat three vegetables at lunch one day, that's okay. If you eat dinner later than usual one night and only end up fasting for eight hours before breakfast, don't worry about it. Your diet will not be derailed, and stressing about it can easily lead to questioning your own self-worth, which is much more difficult to overcome. If the entire plan feels overwhelming, skip to Part III to try to identify and work through the beliefs and thought patterns that are holding you back. For instance, if you are fearful that you will never lose weight and are scared that you have damaged your metabolism from years of unsuccessful dieting, you may find yourself self-sabotaging to prove that you are "right." Unless you reinterpret this false belief to fully accept that you are worthy of getting to your goal weight, it will be challenging to change your habits and behaviors in the long term. But once you've changed this belief, these principles will come so naturally to you that you will rarely eat any other way. You'll have grace and ease around food that you thought eluded you.

CHAPTER 7

Eat Your Vegetables

Plants offer much more than just vitamins, minerals, and fiber. They also contain phytonutrients, plant chemicals that switch on genes that can decrease cellular inflammation and increase the body's ability to clear toxins. Your body needs a variety of fruit and vegetables to function at its most optimal state. If you eat the same salad for lunch day in and day out or avoid certain vegetables and fruits because you've heard they are "inflammatory" or contain too much sugar, you haven't been given the full truth.

First, let's start by clarifying a few food misconceptions:

1. All fruit and vegetables are *anti*-inflammatory, unless you have developed a sensitivity or allergy to one or more of them.
2. All non-starchy vegetables are low in sugar. (I've excluded starchy vegetables like potatoes, sweet potatoes, and yams from this chapter and classified them as carbohydrates in Chapter 10.)
3. Fruit is not a colored lump of sugar. While fruit *does* have more sugar than vegetables, sugar is not the only factor to consider when

determining if something is good for you or not. That's like using the number on the scale to determine your self-worth.

Part of the reason we've become myopically focused on the sugar content of fruit and vegetables is due to the glycemic index (GI), which was developed in 1981 as a way to measure how quickly eating certain carbohydrates causes blood-sugar levels to spike. According to this metric, the lower the body's glycemic response to a food, the healthier it is. The GI index quickly became a popular tool for determining which foods are "better" than others. But the GI discounts the contributions of plant-based phytonutrients, which weren't discovered until the mid-1990s. (Even today only eight thousand phytonutrients have been identified, although scientists estimate there are more than twenty thousand of them in existence.) By the time we started learning about these nutrients, we'd grown accustomed to avoiding foods at the top of the glycemic scale, including carrots, beets, watermelon, and tropical fruits—all of which contain valuable nutrients.

It's worth noting that even the fruits and vegetables that chart higher on the GI contain far less sugar than you may assume once you factor in portion sizes. For instance, 1 cup of pineapple contains only one more gram of sugar than 1 cup of berries. This is equivalent to ¼ teaspoon of sugar. If you've been loading up on berries and avoiding pineapple because pineapple is higher on the GI, you've not only missed out on the pleasure of savoring a juicy slice of pineapple on a sunny summer afternoon but also its unique phytonutrients and enzymes like bromelin, which slow the aging process.

One of the reasons a plant-centric diet supports weight loss is that the phytonutrients trigger the release of gut incretins—gut hormones that improve insulin signaling to decrease fat storage. These incretins also promote the secretion of leptin, a satiety hormone produced by your fat cells. At the same time, the fiber from these plants supports the proliferation of good bacteria such as *Lactobacillus* and *Bifidobacteria*, which convert the fiber into short-chain fatty acids, further stimulating the release of gut satiety incretins. That means, if you want to not be hungry and not store excess body fat, eat your greens—and reds, oranges, yellows, and purples!

A plant's color provides clues to its phytonutrient content and function. I'll explain this in more detail as I go through this chapter, but, in general, the more intense the color, the greater the density of phytonutrients. Color also has certain energetic properties. If you remember your high school physics, you'll recall that each color in the visible light spectrum, from violet to red, is associated with a different wave length and frequency. This frequency has a subtle impact on both the physical body (the body visible to others) and the energetic body (the body invisible to us, which corresponds to our chakras). When you eat fruits and vegetables, their phytonutrients affects your biochemistry and their color frequency affects your energetic body.

In Part I, I provided suggestions on how each of the archetypes could use certain colored plants to support their physical and emotional needs. While you should favor the color that supports your archetype, it's not the only color to eat! And if you feel like one of your chakras (even if it's not the one associated with your archetype) is out of balance, you can eat plants in that color spectrum to help realign yourself. In short: eat as many different types of fruits and vegetables as possible. The more attuned you are to your physical and energetic body, the more you'll notice the subtle changes this dietary guideline brings.

In the Food Fundamentals, I recommended that you eat three different non-starchy vegetables at both lunch and dinner and that these vegetables should make up half of your plate—about 2 to 4 cups. As fruit does contain more sugar than vegetables, limit your consumption to two 1-cup servings per day, as either a snack or part of a meal.

Red Plants

THE PLANTS Heirloom tomatoes, red bell peppers, watermelon, guava, raspberries, cherries, red apples, strawberries, and pomegranates.

THE PHYSICAL The two best-researched phytonutrients in red plants are lycopene and ellagic acid, both of which help protect the skin from sun damage and bones from oxidative stress. In one study, women who consumed 1 tablespoon of tomato paste each day for twelve weeks before being exposed to UV light had lower levels of sun damage compared to those women who didn't eat the tomato paste.[1] In another study, when lycopene was removed from postmenopausal women's diets for four weeks, researchers noticed such a significant change in bone density markers that they concluded that eating a diet without lycopene-rich foods puts women at increased risk of osteoporosis.[2]

THE ENERGETIC Red plants support the root chakra, which represents stability and protection. When the root chakra is out of balance, you can feel isolated and uncertain of your place in the world—like there isn't enough food or money to go around. Nurturers are the most vulnerable to this.

EAT THEM FOR . . . Protection against sunburn; reducing wrinkles and hyperpigmentation; stronger bones; and a deeper connection to your physical environment, peers, and friends.

MENU SUGGESTIONS Strawberry smoothie; tomato and watermelon gazpacho; grilled fish with roasted red peppers; pomegranate in a kale salad; guava as a snack.

PRACTICAL TIP Eat tomato salads before and during a beach vacation and drink watermelon juice while you are poolside to increase the skin's protection against UV light and other free radicals that can cause aging.

Orange Plants

THE PLANTS Carrots, orange bell peppers, apricots, mangoes, nectarines, oranges, clementines, papayas, peaches, gooseberries, cantaloupe, and persimmons.

THE PHYSICAL Orange-pigmented plants are rich in carotenoids such as beta-carotene, alpha-carotene, and zeaxanthin. These phytonutrients help increase skin-cell turnover for a refined and clear complexion. They also boost the immune system by improving the mucosal lining in the nose, throat, and gastrointestinal (GI) tract to decrease bacteria and viruses entering the body.

THE ENERGETIC Orange will bolster the power of the second chakra, the energetic center of beauty and clarity. When the second chakra is out of balance, you can become jealous, judgmental, and restrictive. You may deny yourself pleasure—or overindulge in it. Femme Fatales are the most susceptible to this. (And she's the one avoiding the mango smoothie because she's afraid there's too much sugar in it!)

EAT THEM FOR . . . Clear skin, boosting the immune system, improving mental clarity, dropping judgment, and enhancing self-esteem.

MENU SUGGESTIONS Papaya smoothie; carrot ribbons with mint and pistachios; roasted carrot soup; chia seed pudding topped with fresh apricots; a juicy peach as a snack.

PRACTICAL TIP Drink a papaya smoothie before going on a date to boost your self-confidence.

Yellow Plants

THE PLANTS Golden beets, yellow tomatoes, yellow bell peppers, sweet corn, yellow squash, grapefruit, pineapple, yellow watermelon, lemon, and golden kiwifruit.

THE PHYSICAL Yellow foods contain the phytonutrients lutein and zeaxanthin, which slow the rate of oxidative stress in the body. Decreasing oxidants delays the aging process and frees up the stress hormone cortisol so it can be used to help deal with emotional stressors. These same phytonutrients help prevent macular degeneration by countering free radicals that can damage your eyesight.

THE ENERGETIC The third chakra represents personal identity and yellow plants can help bring it into balance. When the third chakra is out of balance, you can exhibit perfectionist tendencies and become overly controlling and stubborn. Wonder Women are most at risk for a third chakra imbalance.

EAT THEM FOR . . . Reducing stress; bolstering the immune system; enhancing eyesight; increasing mental clarity; and cultivating self-trust, resilience, and dignity.

MENU SUGGESTIONS Golden-beet salad with fresh basil; grapefruit with coconut sugar; yellow bell pepper with hummus; yellow tomatoes drizzled in olive oil with sea salt; snack on golden kiwifruit.

PRACTICAL TIP Eat an omelet with yellow tomatoes before an important business meeting to sharpen your mind and increase your resilience.

RAW VERSUS COOKED

While raw vegetables contain more live enzymes, phytonutrients, and fiber, cooked vegetables are easier to digest, and that may mean you actually get *more* nutrients from them. It's also much easier to eat 1 cup of cooked spinach than 8 cups of raw spinach (the amount needed to make 1 cup of cooked spinach). Contrary to popular belief, heat doesn't destroy vitamins and minerals, but it is true that when you boil vegetables for more than twenty minutes, some of the B vitamins, chlorophyll, and, no doubt, some of the phytonutrients are leached out into the cooking liquid. This is why a slow-cooked stew is so nutritious—you keep all of the good stuff rather than draining it off!

Nonetheless, as soon as you cut a vegetable or fruit, the vitamin C content starts to deteriorate. This is why it's far better to buy whole vegetables than precut ones, though if using precut vegetables is the only way you'll eat them, they're better than nothing!

In general, eat raw vegetables in summer and cooked vegetables in winter. You likely already eat this way since cooked vegetables, stews, and warming broths are more appealing and easier to prepare in winter, while fresh tender greens are more readily available in summer. In the transitional seasons of spring and fall, eat a combination of cooked and raw. However, if you're feeling scattered (hello, Ethereal), skew your meals toward more cooked vegetables, which are very grounding. If you are feeling a little stuck and stagnant, eat more raw vegetables, which help you feel light and airy.

Green Plants

THE PLANTS The deep greens of winter such as kale, Swiss chard, spinach, broccoli, Brussels sprouts, cabbage, and bok choy; spring greens such as gem lettuce, asparagus, celery, cucumber, zucchini, peas, and French beans; fruits such as kiwifruit, pears, green apples, and limes.

THE PHYSICAL Cruciferous vegetables like kale, Brussels sprouts, and Swiss chard contain glucosinolates, which are phytonutrients that alter how estrogen is metabolized. All women benefit from eating cruciferous vegetables, but because Nurturers tend to have excess estrogen, they should include them on a daily basis to help regulate this hormone. Glucosinolates also improve blood-sugar regulation and insulin levels.

Tender greens contain fewer phytonutrients (the ones scientists have identified anyway), but they are still rich in magnesium, vitamin C, manganese, folate, chlorophyll, and potassium. We need all of these nutrients for cellular communication and enzymatic function. Don't skip them.

THE ENERGETIC Green plants support the heart chakra, which is the point of integration between the physical and the intuitive realms. It opens you up to love, kindness, and compassion. When decisions are made under a balanced heart chakra, they are made from unconditional love. If the heart chakra is blocked, love can be transformed into acts of control and manipulation or excluded from your life altogether. By focusing on expanding and opening the heart chakra, you can bring more peace and intimacy into your life. Eating greens can energetically support this. Energetically, the soft spring greens can help to soften you emotionally, while eating earthy greens can help make you more resilient.

EAT THEM FOR . . . Regulating estrogen and insulin levels; reducing the risk of estrogen-sensitive cancers; and opening up to love, kindness, and compassion.

FOOD IDEAS Baby kale in a smoothie; spring green salad with avocado; pea soup with a squeeze of lime; sautéed broccoli rabe with lemon zest.

PRACTICAL TIP If someone has annoyed you, access your compassion by drinking a green juice made of cucumber, lime, green apple, and mint, and forgive them.

Purple Plants

THE PLANTS Purple carrots, eggplant, purple cabbage, blackberries, blueberries, plums, Concord grapes, black figs, dates, cacao, and acai.

THE PHYSICAL These plants are rich in the phytonutrients quercetin, ellagic acid, resveratrol, and anthocyanins, which are most well known for their ability to improve cognition and mental agility. In one study, busy working mothers were asked to drink 12 ounces of Concord grape juice once a day for twelve weeks and then perform a driving test to assess their cognitive function.[3] When they drank the juice, they noticed improvements in their memory and driving performance. Quercetin and resveratrol also have neuroprotective properties and can help regulate chronic inflammation.

THE ENERGETIC The sixth and seventh chakras represent creativity and intuition. Their color frequency is the indigo-violet found in purple plants. When these chakras are out of balance, intuition can be misinterpreted. You can also feel scattered and spacey. Ethereals are governed by these two chakras and are the most vulnerable to these imbalances.

EAT THEM FOR ... Greater brain power; clearer intuition; brain protection; enhancing creativity; integrating intuition with intellect; and feeling grounded and connected.

MENU SUGGESTIONS Roasted vegetable salad with purple carrots; eggplant dip; slaw made with purple cabbage and carrots; fig and cacao truffles.

PRACTICAL TIP If you're feeling scattered, try chia seed pudding topped with cacao nibs and figs.

White Plants

THE PLANTS Onions, leeks, ramps, garlic, scallions, and cauliflower.

THE PHYSICAL Allium, a sulfur compound found in the onion family, acts as an antibacterial and antiviral agent. Cauliflower doesn't contain allium but it does have estrogen- and insulin-regulating glucosinolates, which are also anti-inflammatory and can alter genes that initiate inflammation.

THE ENERGETIC The eighth chakra is located above the head. It is the aura and reflects the well-being of the person projecting it. It is connected with the frequency of white. According to Dharma Singh Khalsa, MD, in *Meditation as Medicine*, "The eighth chakra is the body's first line of defense against illness."[4]

EAT THEM FOR ... Bolstering the immune system; fighting off a bug; enhancing your aura.

FOOD IDEAS Cauliflower topped with hemp seeds; chickpea pancakes with scallions; garlicky lemon vinaigrette; grass-fed steak with ramps; scallions in a kale salad.

PRACTICAL TIP To help fight off a cold, make a warming cauliflower soup with leeks and garlic as soon as you notice symptoms.

CHAPTER 8

The Protein Paradox

We all know that the body needs protein to function properly, but most women don't understand exactly how much they're supposed to eat. In general, women who follow an omnivorous diet tend to *overeat* protein—especially now that protein-rich diets like Paleo and Whole30 have gained traction—while women who follow a vegan diet may not eat *enough*.

If you eat excessive amounts of protein, the most obvious clue is the overdevelopment of muscle, particularly when combined with intense exercise. When Sophia came to me, she complained that her legs looked stocky and bulky. She assumed this was her genetic makeup and feared she'd have to give up her career as a ballerina. Within four weeks, we'd reshaped her legs to look lither and lighter by dramatically recalibrating her protein intake. Kat, a yoga instructor, despaired over her thickset legs, which made her feel more like a shot-putter than a lean yogini. When we cut her protein intake in half and swapped out grass-fed red meat for fish, she rediscovered her lithe physique (and lost twenty-five pounds in the process). This took three months.

While there is an ongoing debate over how much fat or carbs one should consume, protein is the most emotionally charged because it is principally animal based. While there are very real ethical considerations that motivate some people to follow a vegan diet, it's not my place to tell you how to feel about these issues. Instead, I'll focus on the amount and types of protein that are best suited to a female's biochemical needs. Despite what you may have heard, an omnivore diet is no less healthy than a vegan diet, provided you get the composition and quality right. When researchers looked at eleven thousand health-conscious people who ate red meat in addition to raw salads and fresh fruit, they found no difference in cancer, heart disease, or death rates between omnivores and vegetarians.[1] By eating a plant-skewed omnivore diet (which the archetype meal plans are), you'll get the benefit of eating vegetables *and* high-quality protein. If you are a committed vegetarian or vegan, you can still reap the benefits of the Archetype Diet, though because your protein will come from other sources (primarily legumes and grains, which are comprised of more carbs than protein), weight loss might be a little bit slower for you. Just be patient and you'll see results, I promise.

WHY IS PROTEIN IMPORTANT?

Protein is used structurally by the body to create enzymes, neurotransmitters, hormones, skin, bone, muscles, and immune cells. The more metabolically out of balance the body is, the greater the demand for protein. The healthier the body, the less demand for protein. This is why there is no one firm answer on how much protein you should be eating. It depends on the status of your health and your wellness goals. As you read through the seven major functions of protein, think about your body today and whether it requires more protein or less.

The body uses protein in seven important ways:

1. To burn fat: Protein triggers a fat-burning hormone called glucagon, which tells the body to use body fat as its fuel source.

2. To decrease hunger: Protein switches on the gut peptides, which signal to the brain that you're full. This is why it's all too easy to help yourself to a second (or third) slice of bread, but eating a second chicken breast is unappealing.

3. To support the thyroid: The thyroid hormone, thyroxine, is made from the amino acid tyrosine, which is principally found in eggs, turkey, fish, and shellfish.

4. To improve the mood: The neurotransmitters serotonin, dopamine, and GABA (gamma-aminobutyric acid), which biochemically influence our mood, are made from the amino acids tryptophan, tyrosine, and glutamate, respectively.

5. To aid digestion: Digestive enzymes are synthesized from amino acids. If you have insufficient digestive enzymes, you can feel bloated and gassy. Digestive enzymes help break down food into individual components for easy absorption and assimilation.

6. To enhance beauty: The protein molecules collagen, elastin, and keratin are required for thick, luscious hair, firm skin, and strong nails and bones. Protein is also the basis for muscle synthesis. Underdeveloped muscles make the body look fragile.

7. To detoxify the liver: The liver uses amino acids to neutralize toxins so they can be removed from the body safely.

If any of the above cellular processes are a concern for you, you may not be eating enough protein, especially if you're vegan. Temporarily transitioning to a higher-protein diet can be beneficial and help heal the body.

How Much Is Enough?

To enhance weight loss, it's most effective to eat protein at breakfast, lunch, and dinner. Eating protein regularly throughout the day helps to keep blood sugar levels stable, the appetite balanced, and the body in a fat-burning mode. It won't work to double up on protein at dinner—a salad for lunch with no protein and an 8-ounce steak for dinner is not following the plan, even though the total daily protein intake is the same. Beneficial fat-burning hormones are stimulated each time you eat protein, and you'll miss out on these benefits if you don't eat protein regularly.

In general, you can use your palms to guide the amount of protein you should be eating. The larger your body, the larger your palms and the more protein you need to be healthy. For most women, this will be a 4-ounce serving of animal protein at lunch and at dinner, but it may be as small as 3 ounces if you are only five feet tall or up to 5 ounces if you are six feet tall. If you're a Nurturer, you'll add an extra ounce to what you determine your palm size ounce to be. If your palm size indicates 3 ounces, then you'll eat 4 ounces as opposed to the 5 ounces prescribed in the Nurturer chapter. If your palm is equal to 5 ounces, then increase the portion size to 6 ounces.

At breakfast, you'll eat (or drink) 12 to 15 grams of protein. This is equivalent to two eggs or a smoothie made with a plant-based protein powder. You don't need a smoothie with 20 grams or more of protein. More is only better if you are training to be a bodybuilder or a CrossFit champion, but that is a very specific body-shaping goal and beyond the scope of this book.

If you feel hungry all the time, it's likely you are burning up carbohydrates, not body fat. When this happens, it's even more important that you don't feed the body carbohydrates. Instead, eat a larger serving of protein to decrease the appetite and switch the body into a fat-burning mode. Nurturers will benefit the most from increasing their protein intake since they tend to have trouble burning fat. This is why I have added a hint more protein (an extra ounce) to her diet.

You might have noticed that I have not given you an overall protein number to strive for. That's because numbers (calories or grams) distort how you look at food. Instead, focus on a protein-based breakfast and a palm-size serving of protein at lunch and at dinner. Snacks should be fruit, fat, or vegetables and not protein, unless you are looking to develop more muscle or you are diabetic and need extra protein to balance your blood-sugar levels.

NOT ALL PROTEINS ARE CREATED EQUAL

All types of protein will aid in the important bodily functions described above, but there are big differences in the amino acid composition of the various sources of protein. Some, like dairy, stimulate more insulin and decrease fat burning. Others, like grass-fed red meat, contain more leucine and promote muscle synthesis (often needed for the Ethereal). Your archetype's meal plan has been designed with these factors in mind. And while I won't go into the complexities of each protein source, I do want to put the common misconceptions and fears about protein to rest.

Animal-Based Proteins

I want to start by saying that at no point should you be eating meat that has been processed or derived from factory-farmed animals. These have a poor nutritional profile, not to mention severe environmental consequences. The only animal-based proteins I want you to eat are organic, sustainably raised and grass-fed, or wild. If you cannot find these high-quality animal protein choices, please choose a plant protein instead.

THE BEST CHOICE If you want to lose weight and develop toned, elongated muscles, fish and shellfish are by far your best option. When Kat, the yoga instructor who felt like a shot-putter, was tempted to join her husband for a steak, she remembered my guidance: "Fluid, floaty, and feminine." If it glided, it was her energetic match. Instead, she opted for a piece of grilled whitefish drizzled in olive oil, lemon zest, and sea salt. In my group programs, women always lose more weight on those weeks in which they eat mostly seafood rather than other types of animal protein.

Scientists, too, are observing this. In a highly publicized weight-loss study from Israel, researchers studied subjects who followed a high-protein, low-fat diet or a Mediterranean diet for two years. The women on the seafood-rich Mediterranean diet lost the most. In fact, the average weight loss for women on the Mediterranean diet was more than *double* the weight loss of the women on the low-fat and high-protein diets.[2] Interestingly, men lost the most on the meat-heavy, high-protein diet. This is precisely what I see in my practice—men and women respond differently to the same diet.

Why might more fish and less red meat support weight loss? For starters, wild-caught fish have more omega-3s than red meat. Omega-3s help decrease inflammatory mediators that can interfere with fat loss. They also activate genes that can boost the metabolism. In addition, seafood is rich in the thyroid-supporting nutrients selenium and iodine. Without these nutrients, the thyroid cannot perform its metabolism-boosting function. Oily fish such as salmon, tuna, black cod, sardines, and mackerel are most abundant in omega-3s, but even whitefish like halibut, sea bass, lemon sole, cod, and haddock contain them.

But the benefits of eating seafood go way beyond weight loss. The omega-3s, zinc, iron, iodine, and selenium in seafood help with cognition, hormone regulation, antioxidant synthesis, energy, and inhibiting the breakdown of collagen (i.e., reducing wrinkles).

Don't like fish? Shellfish such as octopus, oysters, crustaceans, shrimp, and scallops are also great protein choices. They're particularly rich in zinc, a nutrient that helps stabilize blood-sugar and hormone levels as well as boost mood and attention. Oysters are the richest dietary source of zinc and also contain iron and B12. Six oysters only have 60 calories, fewer than an apple (70 calories or more) and are a smart choice if you eat out often.

One caveat: large fish often contain high levels of mercury. For that reason, you should avoid swordfish, Chilean sea bass, grouper, tilefish, bluefish, king mackerel, ahi tuna, shark, and orange roughy. Albacore and yellowfin tuna have less mercury than ahi tuna because they don't grow to be as large and therefore accumulate less mercury. You may eat albacore and yellowfin tuna up to twice a month, but make sure you eat them with parsley or cilantro, as these herbs help bind up the mercury to safely remove it from the body. You can add these herbs to a salad or top the fish with an herby chimichurri or pesto.

If you want to reduce your risk of mercury intake further, choose smaller fish, such as wild salmon, trout, sea bass, sole, cod, haddock, and sardines. (A full list is included in Appendix A.) Shellfish such as oysters, clams, shrimp, and scallops are also low in mercury. So don't use the fear of mercury as an excuse for avoiding fish entirely. Not eating fish because you're worried about mercury is analogous to eschewing all vegetables because they may have been treated with pesticides; the cognitive, mood, and body-refining benefits of eating these foods outweigh the potential downside, which you can mitigate by making smart choices. Furthermore, recent studies have shown that mercury from fish, which is organic mercury, doesn't have the same neurotoxin effects as mercury from inorganic sources such as dental fillings.[3] Just choose your seafood wisely.

OTHER GOOD OPTIONS After fish, organic eggs are my favorite protein source. They are rich in omega-3s, folate, B12, and choline—all nutrients that support enhanced brain function, a better mood, and greater vitality.[4] Do not be concerned with the cholesterol in the egg yolks. In 2016, researchers announced that, "after sixty years of research, a general consensus has now been reached that dietary cholesterol, chiefly from eggs, exerts a relatively small effect on serum LDL-cholesterol levels and CVD risk."[5] Elevated cholesterol levels are more likely to result from the consumption of excess carbohydrates since carbs convert to cholesterol before going to body fat. As for all animal protein, you should avoid industrialized factory-farmed products. Always choose organic eggs. The serving size is two per meal up to four times per week.

Grass-fed red meat and wild game are also excellent sources of protein as they are rich in iron, zinc, L-carnitine, and B6, all nutrients that support sustainable energy levels. Red meat is the most effective protein source at promoting muscle growth because of its amino acid and fat content. It is, therefore, best suited to the Ethereal, who often has underdeveloped muscles.

If you're worried about the link between red meat and inflammation, heart disease, and cancer, please don't be. Only *processed* red meat like hot dogs, deli meat, salami, and Spam have been associated with these adverse health outcomes. Grass-fed red meat and processed meat have dramatically different nutritional profiles, and putting them into the same category is equivalent to putting a gossipy tabloid magazine alongside an Ernest Hemingway novel and calling it "literature."

Perhaps you've heard that red meat is acidic? Well, so are grains, and this is not a reason to avoid eating them, either. Instead, neutralize that acidic tendency with complementary foods. When you eat red meat or grains with raw salads, fresh herbs, or sautéed vegetables, you alkalize the meal. It's the entirety of the meal you need to consider, not the qualities of any single ingredient in isolation.

A final note: Organic poultry, such as chicken, turkey, duck, and quail, is a decent protein source, but there is nothing nutritionally superior about it. I recommend it as a filler when there are no other suitable protein choices available.

Plant-Based Proteins

Hemp seeds and chia seeds are two of my favorite plant-based proteins because they are not only rich in amino acids but they are low in carbohydrates and contain the hormone-balancing omega-3s and omega-6s.

While I've classified all other seeds as fats (see the next chapter), hemp and chia are rich enough in protein to count as a source, especially if you want a vegan meal. Adding 3 tablespoons of hemp seeds to your vegetable salad will give you the same amount of protein as two eggs. A tabbouleh made with hemp seeds, parsley, mint, tomatoes, and olive oil takes less than three minutes to make and is a complete meal.

Chia seed pudding has been the go-to breakfast among insiders in the wellness community for many years. Three tablespoons of chia seed has the same amount of protein as one egg as well as 12 grams of fiber, the highest amount found in a real food. They are also rich in those skin-beautifying omega-3s. I've included chia seed pudding on all archetype meal plans because chia seeds are such a woman-friendly food.

Plant-based protein powders are a smart way to get protein into the body when you want a lighter form of protein. A pea, rice, and hemp blend is my favorite because this combination decreases the appetite and tastes good. It also improves the composition of the gut microbiome,[6] which is essential for many functions, including energy, detoxification, digestion, and mood. Rice protein doesn't have the same appetite-decreasing properties as pea and hemp protein. If you choose a protein powder made exclusively from rice protein, be warned: you may be hungry an hour later.

All archetypes can consume a plant protein powder up to five times per week. They make an easy and smart breakfast option. Many of my clients have plant-based protein smoothies for breakfast during the week and save eggs for the weekend.

Amino-acid-rich grains and legumes like quinoa, amaranth, lentils, and chickpeas contain more carbs than protein and can slow weight loss in sensitive individuals. As such, I have classified these as carbohydrates and discuss them in more detail in Chapter 10. However, if you follow a vegan diet, it can be very challenging to get enough high-quality protein unless you incorporate these into your meal plan. It is essential, in this case, that you watch your portion size. Keep your servings to no more than ½ cup of cooked grains and legumes at lunch and dinner if you are a

Nurturer, ¾ cup if you are a Femme Fatale or Wonder Woman, or 1 cup if you are an Ethereal, and count this as both your protein and carbohydrate portion.

Proteins to Limit: Dairy and Soy

Industrialized dairy is not the same as cheese and milk from the local farm. It is full of growth hormones and antibiotic residue, both of which have been associated with autoimmune diseases and gut microbiome disruptions. Cheese sticks, ultra-pasteurized milk, and nonorganic yogurt are the Twinkies of the dairy family. They are not worthy of consumption, no matter how much you like the taste.

If, after the four-week dairy hiatus recommended in the Food Fundamentals, you have nasal congestion, allergies, irritable bowel syndrome, acne, or you have an autoimmune condition, I recommend eliminating all dairy for nine full months while simultaneously working on healing your gut lining and microbiome (this is discussed in the Ethereal chapter). After that period, you can then consider reintroducing organic, grass-fed dairy if you desire, following the frequency guidelines suggested for your archetype.

If you're worried that cutting back on dairy will compromise your bone health, don't be. Increasing your intake of green vegetables as well as almonds, hemp seeds, chia seeds, and sesame seeds will give you more bone nutrients than cow's milk. In fact, almond milk has more calcium than cow's milk. Besides, magnesium is even more critical than calcium for bone health because more people are depleted in magnesium than calcium. If you don't have enough magnesium, it will become the rate-limiting step in utilizing the calcium for the bones. Dairy has very low levels of magnesium while greens, almonds, and seeds are rich in both calcium and magnesium.

Organic soy—edamame, tofu, tempeh—is the only soy you should consider eating. The vast majority of the soy in the United States is genetically modified and sprayed with the probable carcinogenic pesticide, glyphosate. But the health debate on soy goes beyond how it is grown. Soy has a weak estrogenic effect on the body, which means it will activate the estrogen receptors in the body. This may be helpful for the Ethereal but worrisome for the Nurturer or anyone else with signs of estrogen dominance. It can also interfere with your thyroid function. Soy consumption must be moderated in accordance with your archetype's guidelines.

Two exceptions are miso and tamari (wheat-free soy sauce), since they are used as a broth or flavor enhancer, not a protein source, and are therefore not consumed in portions large enough to affect hormones.

Bottom line: Protein is critical to a balanced body, but different types will affect your body differently, as will portion sizes. Pay attention to the changes you notice when implementing your meal plan.

CHAPTER 9

Fat Fears and Fetishes

====

Like protein, fat has a structural function in the body. Every single cell membrane is made up of fats—both saturated and unsaturated—which enables the cells to communicate effectively with one another. Dietary fat doesn't convert to body fat if the body needs to use it structurally. If you don't eat the right amount or types of fats, your body and brain go haywire. Too little fat in the body can lead to insulin resistance and weight gain, and this is one of the major drawbacks of the low-fat approach to weight loss. Without enough fat, the integrity of the cell membranes suffers and the body's metabolic processes become distorted because the body can't hear the hormones that tell it to burn fat.

This is very important to understand because the conversion of dietary fat to body fat is not a linear process. The more damaged the cells, the more beneficial fats you need to heal the cell membranes. In addition to building cell membranes, fat is used to build the white and gray matter in the brain, improve memory and mood, keep the skin firm, make hormones, and absorb fat-soluble vitamins. Also, it is the precursor to vitamin D and bile salts. Bile salts help remove toxins, immune debris, and old hormones from the body. They are a crucial part of the body's detoxification process. But if you eat *too* many fats, you may overwhelm the body's ability to emulsify and utilize those fats, causing detoxification issues, hormonal imbalances, acne, and stagnation in the lymphatic system (a fat transportation system).

The body needs both saturated and unsaturated fat. Saturated fat is found primarily in coconut oil, red meat, nuts, cream, cheese, and butter. Unsaturated fat is found in olives, olive oil, avocados, seeds, nuts, and oily fish. Saturated fat is chemically denser than unsaturated fat and helps keep the cell membrane strong and rigid, while unsaturated fat keeps the membrane flexible enough so that nutrients can pass through it. The only "bad" fats are those like trans fats that have been damaged from food processing, and they create hard, impermeable cell membranes.

You should aim to eat a variety of saturated and unsaturated fats. Don't go overboard on one type of fat like coconut oil because it is supposedly "better" for you. (Remember that margarine, with industrialized trans fats, was once consider the "better" fat!) Coconut oil is a good fat but it's not superior to the other fats discussed here.

WHAT FATS TO EAT

Unlike protein and carbs, the serving size for fats differs depending on the type of fat consumed, so pay attention to portions when adding fat to your meals. Note that organic eggs, grass-fed red meat, and fish all contain fats that support the body's biochemical processes, but because they are principally made of protein, that's how I have categorized them. When you eat these foods, you get a protein *with an added fat benefit*, but you do not need to subtract the fat in these foods from your fat allowance.

When choosing a snack, opt for fats over protein or carbs. As explained in the previous chapter, you don't need to eat more protein than what you have at your meals, and carbs can cause your blood sugar to spike without providing the same cell-building benefits as fats. If you opt to snack on avocado, olives, nuts, or seeds, you can double the recommended portion size listed below, provided it remains under your snack caloric limit.

Seeds

Seeds—pumpkin, sunflower, sesame, hemp, chia, and flax—are a woman's food! They are rich in plant-based omega-3s, omega-6s, zinc, magnesium, and manganese. All of these nutrients regulate sex-hormone levels, decrease PMS, decrease perimenopausal symptoms, improve brain function, and prevent the degradation of collagen for ageless skin. Flaxseeds also contain phytoestrogens, which can help regulate estrogen levels, making these highly beneficial for the Ethereal and women in late-stage perimenopause when estrogen starts to decline. Each type of seed has a slightly different nutrient composition, so eat a variety in order to reap their maximum wellness and beauty benefits. Add 1 tablespoon of raw seeds to a green salad, sprinkle 1 tablespoon of sesame seeds over roasted vegetables, or snack on 2 tablespoons of cinnamon-spiced pumpkin seeds.

Nuts

Nuts have more saturated fat and fewer omega-3s and omega-6s than seeds, which makes them chemically and energetically denser. If you feel stuck and stagnant (which is typical for the Nurturer), skip the nuts and eat seeds instead. If you feel scattered, as Ethereals often do, you can eat nuts to feel grounded. Nut butters count as a fat source, but if you can't limit yourself to 1 tablespoon at a time, put them away until you've mastered your mind by working through Part III. I've found that many of my clients have a tendency to overeat nut butters, especially if they are trying to avoid sweets.

The serving size for each type of nut, when used in a meal, is below.

Double these recommendations if you're eating them as a snack. But remember, make sure your snacks are no greater than the caloric limit discussed in Food Fundamental "When Snacking, Calories Matter."

- 8 medium-size nuts like almonds, hazelnuts, walnuts, pecans, and cashews
- 4 macadamia nuts
- 12 shelled pistachios
- 15 pine nuts
- 2 Brazil nuts

The difference in nutrient composition among most types of nuts is relatively insignificant at this portion size, so one nut isn't better than the other. They all contain vitamin E, zinc, manganese, and magnesium. Just go for a variety.

Brazil nuts are one exception. They are the richest dietary source of selenium, which is used for the synthesis of the active thyroid hormone, T3, to boost the metabolism. I recommend that women with a thyroid issue snack on four Brazil nuts several times a week.

Peanuts (which are actually a legume) are often packed in warm, humid silos where they can sweat and grow mold. For this reason, I don't recommend you eat them on a regular basis, but if you're at a restaurant or dinner party and are served peanuts in a salad or as part of a meal, don't pick them out. Not all peanuts have mold, and if you happen to eat some with a smidgen of mold, no big deal—a healthy liver and gut microbiome will eliminate it.

RAW VERSUS ROASTED NUTS AND SEEDS When roasting nuts and seeds, food manufacturers typically use very high temperatures that can damage their delicate fats. If you prefer the crunchy texture of roasted nuts, roast your own at home at a temperature no higher than 375°F. Flaxseeds should only be eaten raw because heat destroys their omega-3s.

Avocado

Avocados are mostly oleic acid, a monounsaturated fat so small it that can slip through the cell membrane and protect the cell's energy-making mitochondria from free-radical damage. When you protect the mitochondria, you slow the aging process. Avocados also contain lutein, zeaxanthin, Coenzyme Q10, and folate. A serving size is ¼ avocado in a meal and ½ avocado as a snack.

Olives and Olive Oil

Extra-virgin olive oil and olives are 75–85 percent oleic acid. They also contain the phytonutrients quercetin and kaempferol, which have antioxidant and anti-inflammatory properties. Beyond olive oil's health benefits, who doesn't love its grassy, citrus-kissed taste? Olives also make a great snack. If you're at a bar that offers roasted nuts and olives as a snack, choose the olives because the nuts are likely to be commercially roasted and their delicate fats damaged. Enjoy up to fifteen olives as a snack or up to eight in a salad.

You may have heard that when you cook with olive oil, its beneficial polyphenols are destroyed. This is only true if the oil is exposed to temperatures above 375°F, so sautéing and roasting are fine, but higher-temperature cooking, such as deep frying, is not. One tablespoon of olive oil is considered a serving, whether you're using it as a dressing or to cook with.

Coconut and Other Oils

Coconut oil has become the new darling of the health-conscious because it is rich in lauric acid, a medium-chain triglyceride (MCT). MCTs are smaller, more soluble saturated fats, which are preferentially used by the cells for energy, making them less susceptible to body fat storage than regular fats, known as long-chain triglycerides. MCTs have also been shown to improve cognition and stabilize synaptic connections in the brain.[1]

Coconut oil also helps to decrease constipation. Add 1 tablespoon to a smoothie in the morning and you'll literally be ready to go! The serving size for coconut oil, as for olive oil, is 1 tablespoon.

Other nut oils like walnut oil, macadamia oil, and hazelnut oil are great alternatives to coconut oil and olive oil. Use these based on your taste preference, knowing that their nutrient profiles are excellent. A serving is 1 tablespoon. Canola, safflower, sunflower, soybean, grapeseed, and peanut oil are often processed with harsh solvents, which damage their omega-3s and omega-6s. If you are going to eat foods that contain these oils, make sure you use organic, unrefined varieties; otherwise skip them.

Grass-fed Butter and Ghee

After your four-week dairy hiatus, you can consider adding grass-fed butter and ghee to your diet, assuming you are not continuing on the dairy hiatus for a full nine months. Ghee is clarified butter and does not contain lactose, casein, or whey, making it safer for people who have a sensitivity to dairy or who are lactose intolerant. Grass-fed butter and ghee contain more butyric acid and conjugated linoleic acid (CLA) than butter from grain-fed cows.[2] Butyric acid supports the proliferation of good gut bacteria and CLA helps to decrease hunger.[3] As with the oils, consider 1 tablespoon a serving.

CHAPTER 10

The Carbohydrate Question

———

Carbs aren't anything to be scared of, but how much you can eat will depend on your metabolism, your level of body fat, and how intensely you exercise. If you have a sluggish metabolism (typical for the Nurturer), high levels of body fat, and you don't exercise often, then you need very few carbs in your diet, particularly if you want to lose weight. However, if you have a relatively fast metabolism, a low level of body fat, and you exercise six or more times a week, then you will absolutely need more carbs. Without them, you'll feel depleted, and those last few pounds you want to get rid of will not come off unless you eat some carbs. Each archetype has an inherent carbohydrate sensitivity, meaning how easily they convert carbs to body fat. The Nurturer is the most sensitive, while the Ethereal is the least sensitive. If this sounds crazy, keep reading— there's science behind all of this.

Carbohydrates are composed of sugars, starches, and cellulose, and unlike protein and fat, they don't have a structural function in the body.

With the exception of fiber, all carbohydrates are metabolized into the sugar molecule, glucose. How quickly these carbohydrates are converted to sugar depends on the amount of fiber, protein, or fat the food (or meal) contains. The more fiber, protein, or fat you consume along with your carbs, the more slowly glucose will be released into the blood. This is why legumes, which are rich in fiber and protein, have a slower glucose response than white bread.

Once converted, these glucose molecules need to go somewhere in the body. The three options are blood sugar, glycogen (stored energy), and body fat. The hormone insulin directs the storage of glucose to glycogen or body fat. It tells the muscle and liver cells to open up and store glucose as glycogen or the fat cells to store glucose as triglycerides. When insulin is elevated due to excess glucose in the body, it's physically impossible for the body to burn body fat because insulin tells the body to *store* fat and not burn it.

If the body is functioning properly, the glucose storage process is relatively linear, with body fat being stored only after the glycogen stores are full. This is not the case if you have chronically elevated insulin levels. This is known as insulin resistance and is a precursor to type 2 diabetes. When this happens, the cells become overwhelmed by insulin and stop responding—much in the way you shut down when someone starts screaming at you. Under these conditions, the body preferentially stores glucose as body fat, not glycogen. The muscle and liver cells don't absorb the level of glucose they once did, which means you have less glucose available for energy but more available for fat storage. This is why you can eat carbs, not feel energized, and gain weight. The energy stores have closed their doors, but the fat cells are wide open for business. Overweight Nurturers tend to be insulin resistant, which is why they should consume fewer carbohydrates than the other archetypes.

Fortunately, Nurturers can reverse insulin resistance by dramatically decreasing the starchy carbohydrates in their diets and adding in the healing nutrients discussed in Step 3 of their program. When the cells have resensitized to insulin, the amount of insulin needed to manage glucose properly is reduced significantly and fat storage decreases dramatically.

WHAT CARBS TO EAT

This category encompasses legumes, grains, and starchy vegetables. For the purpose of menu planning, I am distinguishing starchy vegetables from the fruits and vegetables covered in Chapter 7. Although those items also contain carbohydrates, they contain relatively few carbohydrate molecules and so do not need to be counted as part of your carbohydrate allowance. Carb-heavy foods like cakes, cookies, cereals, breads, and pastries contain few nutrients and should be an occasional treat, not part of your day-to-day meals. The only "bad" carbs I want you to avoid entirely are those that have been highly processed and damaged by our industrial food system; these include prepackaged cookies, crackers, and cakes, potato chips and pretzels, sugary cereals, and white bread.

Because different body types process carbohydrates in different ways, the amount you should consume will depend on your archetype, but, ultimately, only you will be able to determine the amount that is right for you. The amount of starchy carbs you eat will depend on your body-shaping goals, how sensitive you are to carbs, and the duration and intensity of your exercise. If you are trying to lose weight, you should eat fewer carbs than if you are eating for maintenance. If you exercise intensely for more than five hours a week, you may add an extra ½ cup of starchy carbs to your archetype's lunch and dinner base serving for every hour in excess of the five that you work out. These extra carbs will help you store much-needed energy so you don't feel tapped out from your workouts.

The recommended serving size is the same no matter which carbohydrate you choose; ½ cup of beans is the same as ½ cup of rice. There are, however, some subtle differences I want you to be aware of that might influence your choice. Legumes such as lentils, chickpeas, black beans, cannellini beans, and red kidney beans contain the highest levels of protein and fiber. They are approximately one-third protein, one-third fiber, and one-third net carbs. (Net carbs are carbs that will be converted to glucose for energy or fat storage. Fiber is a carb that *isn't* converted to glucose, so it does not count as a net carb. Instead, it's used as fuel by the gut bacteria.)

If you've ever tried the Paleo diet, you'll know there's concern in that community that legumes and grains contain naturally occurring proteins called lectins and phytates that can damage the lining of the GI tract and act as anti-nutrients. However, lectins are mostly deactivated by soaking and cooking, and since the vast majority of legumes and grains are cooked (who eats raw lentils?) or soaked if you're following a raw diet (sprouted hummus, yes please!), this is an ill-conceived argument.

It's true that phytates can bind to minerals and inhibit the absorption of zinc and iron in foods, but your gut bacteria break down phytates. Phytates have also been shown to clear heavy metals from the body as well as decrease free radicals. Rather than being an anti-nutrient, they can be a protective compound. I hold a very simple view: Plants are beneficial. If they contain components that are reputedly not good for you, other components will offset them. You want to look at the synergy of the entire plant, not individual nutrients or anti-nutrients.

If you get bloated or gassy when you eat legumes, it's not the legumes' fault. Humans don't have the enzymes to break down the fiber in legumes, but the microflora in our guts do! If bloat is a problem, it's possible that the good bacteria in your gut have been depleted or damaged, so get to work on restoring your gut microbiome (see Chapter 5 on the Ethereal for more on this) and you'll be able to eat these highly beneficial legumes without discomfort.

A sampling of my favorite meals containing legumes are a black lentil and beet salad; chickpeas and vegetable soup; cannellini beans with avocado and carrots wrapped in lettuce leaves; and black beans with micro greens and roasted carrots.

Grains, such as rice, wheat, oats, millet, and maize, and pseudograins, like quinoa, buckwheat, teff, and amaranth, have less protein than legumes, but they are still an excellent source of amino acids as well as vitamin B6, which helps regulate the sex hormones and create neurotransmitters, the chemical messengers that influence our mood. They are also rich in fiber, magnesium, and manganese—three nutrients that help stabilize blood-sugar levels. The grains also contain anti-inflammatory phytonutrients such as quercetin, rutin, and flavonoids. You can add a sprinkling of purple wild rice over your green salad, add quinoa to an organic chicken and vegetable soup, or use soba noodles as a base for wild salmon and wok-tossed greens. If you have an autoimmune disease, I recommend avoiding all grains (gluten-free or otherwise) because grains can damage your fragile digestive tract.

The final type of carb I recommend are starchy vegetables, including sweet potatoes, new potatoes, purple potatoes, winter squash, turnips, yams, and parsnips. These contain very few amino acids, but they are, like all vegetables, rich in phytonutrients. Some of my personal favorites are a warm vegetable salad of purple potatoes, sweet potato frittata, roasted butternut squash on a green salad, or sliced yam with coconut oil. Choose your starchy vegetables based on your taste preference and its color, which reflects the phytonutrients and the chakra-rebalancing properties discussed in Chapter 7.

THE DIGEST ON GLUTEN

Given the hysteria surrounding gluten, it's easy to question whether this is just the latest health fad or a real issue affecting our bodies. The earliest documentation of what we now call celiac disease was recorded in the first century by a Greek physician, though it wasn't until the twentieth century that scientists identified gluten as the culprit.[1] However, in the past fifty years, thanks to the rapid industrialization of our food system, gluten intolerance has been on the rise.

In the late 1960s, wheat was crossbred, hybridized, and reengineered to increase its yield. This alteration deliberately increased the molecular size of gluten so that bread would rise and become more elastic and chewy. However, gluten is a protein and changing the size of a protein molecule leads to its own set of health ramifications, just like changing the serving size of soda from 8 ounces to 32 ounces does.

In addition to those changes, in 1974 Monsanto patented its herbicide Roundup, a weed killer, for use on crops including wheat, oats, corn, and soy. Roundup contains glyphosate, which Dr. Stephanie Seneff at the Massachusetts Institute of Technology has linked to "leaky gut," an altered microbiome, and increases in autism.[2] In 2015, the World Health Organization's cancer group, the International Agency for Research on Cancer, classified glyphosate as a probable carcinogen. Add to this eating on the run, eating quickly, and high stress levels (all of which decrease the enzymes needed to digest gluten), as well as an altered gut microbiome from processed food and antibiotics, and the stage has been set for a hyperimmune reaction to gluten.

As recommended in the Food Fundamentals, during the first four weeks on your archetype plan, exclude wheat, barley, oats, and rye, which all contain gluten, from your diet. Don't eat *anything* made with flour, including a bite of your friend's avocado toast, gourmet pizza, homemade pasta, or freshly baked cookies. Watch out for wheat hidden in soy sauce, oyster sauce, hoisin sauce, and teriyaki sauce. Remember, it's just four weeks.

If you have any of the symptoms listed below and they return when you reintroduce gluten after four weeks, consider committing to a nine-month gluten hiatus to help rebalance the body.

- Your weight fluctuates by five pounds over several days.[3]
- You have insulin resistance.[4]
- You feel fatigued and spacey.[5]
- Your stomach is perpetually bloated.[6]
- You get hangry (angry when hungry).
- You have eczema or psoriasis.[7]
- You have unexplained diarrhea.[8]
- You feel depressed, anxious or manic.[9]
- Your joints ache.[10]

When you reintroduce gluten, choose heirloom grains like organic spelt, farro, einkorn, and kamut because their gluten molecule is smaller and less reactive than those of other gluten-containing grains. Organic sourdough is traditionally fermented and made with only organic wheat, sea salt, water, and naturally occurring yeast. The fermentation helps break down the gluten molecule to a smaller molecule so that it is less reactive. Research is now emerging that even some celiacs can tolerate bread that has been made using traditional fermentation methods.[11] Aim to keep your consumption of wheat, rye, oats, or barley to no more than once a week after the hiatus.

A note about gluten-free substitutes: Since gluten is a protein, it slows the glycemic response. When processed foods replace gluten sources with pulverized corn, rice, and potato starch, these packaged goods will spike your blood sugar far more dramatically than gluten-containing carbs. In a nutshell: they are junky substitutes. You're better off eating the whole starchy carb these substitutes are made from instead. For example, a salad with whole chickpeas is a better choice than a slice of gluten-free bread made with chickpea flour. Similarly, roasted potatoes are better than a slice of gluten-free bread made with potato starch.

However, there are times when all you want is avocado toast, and if you're following a gluten-free plan, gluten-free bread is your "I'm not missing out" option. Look for gluten-free options that are made with more protein-dense grains like quinoa, millet, and brown rice. You can consider these part of your starchy carb allowance on your archetype eating plan.

CHAPTER 11

The Seduction of Sugar

I n my experience, there are five types of sugar eaters: 1) the reward eater who eats dark chocolate as a treat for making it through the day; 2) the comfort eater who soothes herself with ice cream or a blueberry muffin; 3) the mindless eater who grabs handfuls of M&M's from the office candy bowl without thinking twice about it; 4) the habitual eater who needs dessert every night because she hasn't gone without it for years; and 5) the final type, the addicted eater, who goes into a tailspin of anxiety at the thought of giving up sweets.

Wonder Women tend to be reward eaters, while Nurturers tend to comfort-eat, but these sugar-eating patterns transcend the archetypes, and, depending on your mood or situation, you can be any of the above. The first four are psychological behaviors, while the addicted eater is bio-chemically and psychologically wired to crave sugar. This chapter dis-cusses the biochemical reasons for sugar cravings, though in Part III I will explore the psychological reasons behind why you can't seem to quit sugar.

Sugar, when eaten in excess, not only slows weight loss but can also trigger hormonal imbalances, promote the proliferation of pathogenic microbes in the gut, create wrinkles, exacerbate inflammation, make you crave even more sugar, make you hungry, and increase your risk for diabetes, obesity, and cancer. It can also affect your mood by destabilizing the brain chemistry, making you feel depressed or anxious. In essence, sugar can steal your beauty, brains, and brilliance, but it all depends on how much you consume. A couple of teaspoons of sugar a day are not going to turn you into a moody bitch with wrinkles, inflammation, and fat thighs. If you need a hint of sugar to satisfy a craving that would otherwise have you reaching for cakes, cookies, and ice cream, you're permitted.

My three favorite sugars are coconut sugar, raw honey, and maple syrup because they give you a hint of sweetness while providing minerals such as magnesium and potassium (and in the case of raw honey, prebiotics for your gut microflora). Use these sugars based on taste preference, not on glycemic response. You should be using them in such small amounts that you won't need to worry about the effect on your blood-sugar levels.

The caveat: if you find yourself drinking from the maple syrup bottle or going through a jar of raw honey in three days, keep them out of your diet until you've changed the biochemical imbalance that is causing this obsessive behavior. Don't worry, you're not a glutton. There is something going on biochemically, and we'll get to that.

NOT ALL SUGARS ARE CREATED EQUAL

Sugar, as in table sugar, is approximately 50 percent glucose and 50 percent fructose. While fructose gets a bad rap, it's not necessarily the devil it's made out to be. The body is designed to tolerate a small amount of fructose. In fact, we have specific fructose receptors on the lining of the small intestine that transport fructose into the cells. However, there's a limit to how much fructose the cells can absorb. When they are full, the excess fructose goes straight to the liver, where it can cause fatty liver, or to your belly, where it is converted into visceral fat[1] (i.e., the hard belly fat that produces inflammatory substances). This is why you want to avoid large doses of fructose but you don't need to be frightened of fruit. The amount of sugar in a moderate portion of fruit (about 1 cup) isn't enough to saturate the cells with fructose; just don't sit down to a large fruit platter reminiscent of those popularized in the late 1980s spa diets! Excess fructose is not good, no matter the source.

Fructose should not be confused with high-fructose corn syrup (HFCS). HFCS has the same glucose and fructose percentage as table sugar, but it is made from genetically modified corn sprayed with glyphosate. It is used in many sugar-sweetened beverages like soda, fruit juice, sports drinks, and energy drinks. Sugar, such as HFCS, consumed in a liquid form is the most damaging to the body and brain because it bypasses the appetite-suppressing hormones, which are activated when you chew.[1] Drinking sugar increases the risk of obesity and insulin resistance, not to mention fatty liver and visceral fat because beverages don't contain other ingredients, like fat and flour, which trigger the release of appetite-suppressing hormones to tell the body you are full. So while a serving of cake may contain the same amount of sugar as a serving of soda, you'll typically consume less food later on in the day if you eat the cake versus drinking a soda. A piece of cake may become lunch; a soda never will. Sadly, we're seeing six-year-old kids with fatty liver disease because they drink soda like water (one of my clients was actually bottle-fed cola!). There's no good reason why soda (or other forms of liquid sugar) should be in your diet. The same applies to HFCS. Nix it now.

Diet soda isn't any better than the "real" stuff. The fake, calorie-free sweeteners added to diet drinks change the gut microbiome for the worse, trigger insulin, and are highly addictive.[2] If you're addicted to soda (diet or otherwise), try replacing it with kombucha, a fizzy, fermented tea that comes in many different flavors and is actually good for you, as it can help repopulate the gut microbiome with beneficial microbes that support weight loss.

A note on agave. Agave can be 50 to 90 percent fructose. You don't need to be concerned about the fructose percentage if you're just stirring a teaspoon into your tea. If, however, you're making a cake with it and you're going to eat the entire thing (I know some of you), then the higher percentage of fructose found in agave is an issue. Swap it out for maple syrup or coconut syrup, which have much lower percentages of fructose.

IS SUGAR ADDICTIVE?

When I was in my mid-thirties, I developed an almost-nightly ritual of making cacao truffles at ten p.m. I felt viscerally pulled toward the kitchen, where I found myself rolling a mixture of cacao, coconut oil, dates, and almonds into balls—and then eating most of the truffles on the spot! The kitchen became a place of fear. If you've never experienced this magnetic pull toward food, you may not understand this, but if you have, you get it, that pain of not feeling like you can trust yourself. Rationally, I absolutely did not want to create those treats, but there was a power beyond my consciousness that drove me to make them anyway. And it wasn't because I had a magnesium deficiency that was making me crave cacao and almonds (a common justification I hear for eating chocolate).

Eating sugar (and even the very thought of it) triggers the release of the pleasure neurotransmitter dopamine. But just because sugar stimulates dopamine and triggers the same brain circuitry as recreational drugs doesn't mean it *is* a drug. Meditation, connection, intimacy, sex, yoga, breath work, trying new foods, and exercise can also release dopamine, but we're not necessarily addicted to them. For a substance to be addictive, it also needs to induce behavioral changes like bingeing, withdrawal, craving, and tolerance. If you feel like you're addicted to sugar, you're likely to believe that sugar can make you act this way, but before you tag yourself as a sugar addict, ask yourself whether you are addicted to other foods like nut butters, popcorn, crackers, or the opulence of eating. If so, it may not be sugar that is addictive but rather *eating* that is addictive for you. That is more psychological than physical because the "addiction" applies to foods beyond sugar.

Researchers aren't convinced that sugar is addictive, either.[3] Many of the headlines proclaiming things like "Sugar is more addictive than cocaine!" actually misinterpret the studies cited. In one case, researchers found that rats could become addicted to saccharine, the noncaloric sweetener found in Sweet'N Low, but sugar was proclaimed to be addictive, not the sugar substitute.[4] Other research shows that when rats are deprived of their food, they gorge on sugar,[5] but when their food isn't restricted, they don't binge on sweets.[6] As any woman on a diet knows, chocolate is never more appealing than when she can't have it.

In order for someone to be classified as an addict, they must show symptoms of withdrawal. Most women aren't going into the kitchen to pour packets of granulated sugar down their throats, nor are they behaving like junkies looking for their next hit. They may have anxiety-filled, sleepless nights and be testy for a week as they settle into not getting what they want, but that's the extent of it.

WHY YOU MIGHT *REALLY* BE CRAVING SUGAR

If sugar isn't addictive, what might be causing your cravings? There are many reasons that could be at work:

You want a feel-good dopamine hit. Indeed, sugar gives you that, but so do pleasurable noneating activities like intimacy, sex, meditation, group exercise, conscious breathing, going to the movies, and dancing. And unlike sugar, these activities provide a lingering high because they also produce oxytocin and serotonin—two well-known happiness-delivering brain chemicals.

Interestingly, when researchers made rats' cages more fun by adding toys such as hamster wheels and plastic igloos and improving the overall environment (they went from a one-level cage to a triplex), they discovered the rats consumed 90 percent less sugar.[7] All the rats needed was a pleasurable distraction and a prettier home and they no longer felt drawn to the sweet food.

Researchers also found that breast-feeding soothed newborns more effectively than giving them droplets of sugar water.[8] Not only is the breast milk nourishing, but the skin-to-skin contact between the baby and its mother releases oxytocin and dopamine, which calms infants and adults alike.[9]

Another way to alter the brain chemistry is through meditation. Meditation has consistently been shown to increase activity in the prefrontal cortex, which improves self-control and rational thought. Addiction short-circuits communication to the prefrontal cortex but meditation rewires it. If you feel you have a dependency on sweet foods, meditation *must* be part of your recovery program. Group meditation is even more powerful because you get the added oxytocin from being connected to the group.

You haven't slept. Without a doubt, if you don't sleep well or get less than 6.5 hours of sleep in a night, you'll crave more sugar and fat-dense food because the lack of sleep can change the appetite-regulating hormones ghrelin and leptin. The solution isn't to eat sweets, it's to get more sleep! We'll talk more about the benefits of a good night's sleep in Part III.

You've skipped meals. When your blood sugar drops too low, even your kid's slobbered-on candy looks enticing. But while your brain might be screaming at you to go for the sugar hit, what your physical body really wants is a nutrient-dense meal. Before you reach for the candy, pause, breathe, and prepare yourself a meal. Sit down to eat it. Vow to make time for yourself. Eating shouldn't be a last-minute consideration. It's crucial to your health, brain, and mood. Structure your day to allow time for three regular meals.

You've got PMS. Don't fight it. Instead of laying into that brownie, though, increase your starchy carbs. Make a frittata with baby potatoes, zucchini, and tomatoes or have black bean pasta with tomatoes, basil, and vegetables. If you're certain you're about to get your period that day, have some dark chocolate. It will be part of your pleasure meal.

You have food sensitivities. When you crave sugar, you are usually craving the sweet-fat combination found in cookies, cakes, chocolate, ice cream, and pastries. That's why a brownie trumps fruit for dessert. What do these foods have in common? They're attached to gluten and dairy, two of the most common food sensitivities.

Food sensitivities can alter the brain chemistry and depress serotonin levels, as the serotonin is sequestered to counter the inflammation those sensitivities cause. When serotonin levels are low, you'll crave more sugary foods, as they are the quickest (but not the most effective) way to increase serotonin. Eliminating gluten and dairy from your diet allows your brain serotonin levels to rise naturally, as you have access to all the serotonin your brain synthesizes.

Your last meal was too salty. If you crave something sweet immediately after a meal, your meal may have been too salty. A balanced flavor contains fat, acid, salt, and sweet, FASS for short. If one element is overly dominant, you'll crave the flavor that was submissive in the meal, most commonly the sweetener. The antidote for this is not sugar but water to dilute the saltiness. Have a glass of sparkling mineral water instead of dessert.

Your brain is playing tricks on you. In Part III, we'll delve more deeply into how to counteract the psychological hooks that keep leading you back to sugary (and other) foods, but for now I want to say that once you reevaluate the psychological reasons that cause you to overeat, you will find it much easier to let go of the cravings that dominate your behavior. With time, the cravings will go away for good!

One evening when I was in my compulsive-chocolate-truffle-making phase, I thought hard about why I continued to make myself sweets when eating them only made me feel terrible and disappointed with myself afterward. I realized I was nurturing myself with those treats. This shouldn't have been a surprise; that was one of the ways my own mother showed affection—dessert every night! Once I saw the association, it was an easy fix. I decided to make the Wonder Woman's tea. A cup of warm tea is very nurturing for me, and something my mother also did for me. In an instant, my desire to continually whip up sweets vanished.

And that's my final point on sugar and addiction: *Your thoughts are more powerful than any sugar-triggered dopamine release from the brain.* You are not powerless before sweets; they do not control you.

CHAPTER 12

Permission for Pleasure

═════

Pleasure makes us feel alive. Without it, a woman can become a distorted version of herself. When we are too busy, too fearful, or too consumed with what others think of us or need from us, we can turn to food as a substitute for the pleasure we are missing in other parts of our lives. As Jungian analyst Marion Woodman describes, "the longing for sweets is really a yearning for love or sweetness."

Your treat meals are essential for developing a long-term relationship with food. Restriction is on the same spectrum as compulsion; both are behaviors that come from lack of trust in yourself. Because of this, about 30 percent of women I work with initially don't want to add the treat meals because they worry that doing so will trigger an insatiable craving for more carbs and fat. I allow them to do this for the first four weeks, then I am much more insistent about them adding the treat meal into their weekly plan.

A case in point: Suzy was 170 pounds when she came to see me. At five foot one, she was obese. She did not eat a single starchy carb or treat for nine months. She achieved her goal of 108 pounds and maintained this weight for about three years. Then . . . she put it all back on—a sad and all-too-common story. Suzy hadn't created a harmonious relationship with food. She still feared it.

As part of the Food Fundamentals, I propose one treat meal or snack—something that feeds your feminine soul—each week. It could be coconut ice cream on a lazy summer afternoon, six squares of dark chocolate and a cognac by the fireplace, or truffle fries and mezcal as you giggle with your best friend about your dating mishaps or your partner's annoying habits. These treats are for enjoyment, and that, in itself, is a form of nourishment. There's a profound difference between diving into a plate of fig-and-almond cookies and immediately feeling guilty about it versus putting the cookies on a pretty plate, playing soft music, and savoring the hints of cardamom, honey, and figs as you taste each bite. It's the same food, but the intention—compulsion vs. pleasure—couldn't be more disparate.

There's no restriction on what you eat, but this isn't a binge fest. It's not pizza and beer followed by Skinny Cow ice cream at a friend's party because there was nothing else to eat. It's not a "cheat" day or even a "cheat" meal. It's a treat *and it's for pleasure.*

Treat meals can also consist of healthy foods that are not on your archetype's meal plan because they contain too many carbohydrates for daily consumption. For instance, you might enjoy avocado on gluten-free toast, granola with coconut yogurt, or a macrobiotic bowl with squash, rice, and beans. If lasagna is one of your favorite dishes, you can have it provided you're not abstaining from gluten and dairy. (The treat meals should *only* contain gluten and dairy if you're absolutely sure you don't have a sensitivity to these foods.)

WHAT ABOUT PORTION SIZES?

There's no limit on portion sizes for your treat meals because I want you to have the freedom to let go of any rules around food. If you want a big bowl of pasta accompanied by a glass of red wine followed by tiramisu, go for it. But the treat meal should never feel obsessive. I had one client who approached her treat meal much as an addict would her drug of choice, planning in advance exactly what she was going to have. She'd dream about it and then, when it finally came time to have her treat meals, she was like a caged animal that had been released.

When we delved into the psychology behind this behavior, we discovered that my client's parents hadn't allowed sweets in the house when she was a kid. She would buy them in secret with her pocket money and eat them under the bed covers. Her beloved grandmother, whom she visited weekly, would also give her a little stash of sweets to take home with her. When her mother discovered the candy wrappers under her bed, she cut off her pocket money and forbade her seeing her grandmother for three months.

She had learned to associate sweets with secrecy and punishment, so when I gave her permission to eat the treats, she tried to get as much in before anyone stopped her again. It was only when we teased out this memory and released her unconscious fear of being shamed and disconnected that she was finally able to create peace with food again.

WHAT ABOUT ALCOHOL?

Your limit is four glasses of alcohol per week. If you're not a drinker, this will feel generous; if you are, this can feel oppressive. But trust me, you will still feel connected and have a life with four or fewer glasses per week. You're just not used to it . . . yet! If you're using alcohol as permission to switch off—a Wonder Woman habit—skip to Chapter 20 for alternative ways to address this.

The best alcohol choices are organic wine, organic champagne, tequila, mezcal, gin, and gluten-free (not grain-based) vodka, as these contain fewer sugars and carbs than beer and brown spirits like rum and whiskey.

Drink only organic wine and champagne, as nonorganic varieties may be made from grapes that were sprayed with pesticides and yeast that has been genetically modified.

Tequila, mezcal, vodka, and gin have less sugar than wine but not by much. The difference between a 2-ounce shot of tequila and a 5-ounce glass of wine is ¼ teaspoon of sugar, so you can choose your drink of choice based on your preference. Clear liquor is *only* better than wine if you are very sensitive to sugar. If you feel excessively hungover or experience nasal stuffiness after drinking one glass of wine, but are drinking nonorganic wine, your symptoms could be from the additives, the genetically modified yeast, or pesticide residue on the grapes rather than an inherent sensitivity. You might also have an overgrowth of *Candida* in your gut that is triggering these symptoms. Chapter 5 explains how to clear Candida from the gut and restore the gut microbiome. Beer contains gluten and yeast, so if you want a flat stomach, skip it.

While abstinence works for substance abuse, food is essential to your very existence and you must learn to create a trusting relationship with it. Only by eating your own birthday cake or the occasional piece of blueberry pie will you come to understand that doing so doesn't automatically lead to weight gain or turn you into a sugar addict.

CHAPTER 13

Archetype Meal Plans

———

I've designed each archetype's meal plan to follow the guidelines outlined in Part I. All of the recipes are included in the next chapter, though there are countless other meals and snacks you can eat on the Archetype Diet. I suggest starting with your archetype's meal plan for the first ten days so you can experience how good it feels to eat this way.

NURTURER MEAL PLAN

	DAY 1	DAY 2	DAY 3	DAY 4	DAY 5
BREAKFAST	Cherry Chocolate Smoothie	Strawberry Hemp Smoothie	Matcha Avocado Smoothie	Golden Smoothie Bowl	Chia Seed Pudding with Raspberries
LUNCH	Pan-Roasted Wild Salmon with Beet and Spinach Salad	Smoked Trout and Vegetable Plate with Hemp and Chia Pesto	Shrimp and Veggie Avocado Bowl	Salmon Burger with Salsa	Tomato and Watermelon Gazpacho Topped with Crab
SNACK	Fresh Blueberries	Pink Mylk	4 Brazil Nuts with Goji Berries	Nori with Carrot Turmeric Hummus and Avocado	Nori with 1/2 Avocado
DINNER	Pan-Seared Lemon Sole with Wild Arugula Salad	Halibut with Curried Vegetables and Potato	Seared Scallops over Cauliflower Puree with Moroccan Carrot Salad	Hemp-Crusted Mahi Mahi with Roasted Vegetables	Cajun Fish Tacos with Summer Slaw
SNACK	Ruby Red Grapefruit with Caramelized Coconut Sugar	Berry-Mint Salad	8oz Kombucha	Two Fresh Figs with 4 Almonds	1 Coconut Macaroon

DAY 6	DAY 7	DAY 8	DAY 9	DAY 10	
Soft-Boiled Eggs with Grape Tomatoes	Tomato and Zucchini Omelet	Pink Smoothie Bowl	Scarlet Red Smoothie	Chia Seed Pudding with Fresh Apricots	**BREAKFAST**
Chicken and Vegetable Soup	Turmeric Chicken with an Israeli Salad	Roasted Cauliflower with Chicken in a Tahini Dressing	Cod and Summer Squash Pasta with Green Goddess Dressing	Smoked Wild Salmon with Kale and Fennel Salad	**LUNCH**
Cinnamon-Spiced Pumpkin Seeds	Watermelon Slices	Avocado with Cumin	Miso Soup	Green Vegetable Juice	**SNACK**
Grilled Shrimp with Cucumber Dill Salad	Treat Meal	Sautéed Cod over Ratatouille	Cauliflower Rice Bowl	Turkey Meatballs with Herbed Salad	**DINNER**
1 cup Fresh Strawberries	1 cup Fresh Raspberries	2 Brazil Nuts Dipped in 2 teaspoons Tahini with Cinnamon	1 cup Watermelon Slices	1 cup Blackberries	**SNACK**

WONDER WOMAN MEAL PLAN

	DAY 1	DAY 2	DAY 3	DAY 4	DAY 5
BREAKFAST	Pineapple Green Smoothie	Green Detox Smoothie	Matcha Avocado Smoothie	Golden Smoothie Bowl	Chia Seed Pudding with Golden Kiwifruit
LUNCH	Mediterranean Salmon Salad	Smoked Trout and Vegetable Plate with Hemp and Chia Pesto	Shrimp and Veggie Avocado Bowl	Turkey Burger with Salsa	Turmeric Chicken with Quinoa and Israeli Salad
SNACK	Pink Grape-fruit with Caramelized Coconut Sugar	Matcha Green Mylk	Fresh Papaya with Lime	Nori with Carrot Turmeric Hummus and Avocado	16 Raw Almonds
DINNER	Pan-Seared Lemon Sole with Wild Arugula Salad	Halibut with Curried Vegetables and Potato	Seared Scallops over Sweet Pea Puree with Moroccan Carrot Salad	Hemp-Crusted Mahi Mahi with Roasted Vegetables	Cajun Fish Tacos with Summer Slaw
SNACK	24 Pistachios	Citrus-Mint Salad	8oz Kombucha	Two Dried Figs with 4 Almonds	1 Coconut Macaroon

DAY 6	DAY 7	DAY 8	DAY 9	DAY 10	
Soft-Boiled Eggs with Yellow Tomatoes	Tomato and Zucchini Omelet	Blue Smoothie Bowl	Kiwi Smoothie	Chia Seed Pudding with Dried Apricots	**BREAKFAST**
Tomato and Watermelon Gazpacho Topped with Crab	Lemony Lentil Soup	Roasted Cauliflower and Squash Salad with Chicken	Cod and Summer Squash Pasta with Green Goddess Dressing	Smoked Wild Salmon with Spring Salad	**LUNCH**
Cinnamon-Spiced Pumpkin Seeds	Fresh Raspberries	4 Black Sesame Seed Crackers	Miso Soup	Green Vegetable Juice	**SNACK**
Pan-Seared Steak with Cucumber Dill Salad	Treat Meal	Sautéed Cod over Ratatouille	Lamb Meatballs with Herbed Salad	Cauliflower Rice Bowl	**DINNER**
1 cup Pineapple Slices	Pink Grape-fruit with Caramelized Coconut Sugar	2 Fig and Coconut Balls	1 cup Watermelon Slices	2 Brazil Nuts Dipped in 2 teaspoons Tahini with Cinnamon	**SNACK**

FEMME FATALE'S MEAL PLAN

	DAY 1	DAY 2	DAY 3	DAY 4	DAY 5
BREAKFAST	Papaya Coconut Smoothie	Ginger Mango Smoothie	Matcha Avocado Smoothie	Golden Smoothie Bowl	Chia Seed Pudding with Fresh Peaches
LUNCH	Mediterranean Salmon Salad	Smoked Trout and Vegetable Plate with Hemp and Chia Pesto	Shrimp and Veggie Avocado Bowl	Turkey Burger with Salsa	Turmeric Chicken with Quinoa and Israeli Salad
SNACK	2 Nectarines	Golden Mylk	Fresh Papaya with Lime	Nori with Carrot Turmeric Hummus and Avocado	Orange Bell Pepper Slices with 2 tablespoons Carrot Turmeric Hummus
DINNER	Pan-Seared Lemon Sole with Wild Arugula Salad	Halibut with Curried Vegetables and Potato	Seared Scallops over Sweet Pea Puree with Moroccan Carrot Salad	Hemp-Crusted Mahi Mahi with Roasted Vegetables	Cajun Fish Tacos with Summer Slaw
SNACK	16 Raw Hazelnuts	Pink Grapefruit with Caramelized Coconut Sugar	8oz Kombucha	Two Fresh Figs with 4 Almonds	1 Coconut Macaroon

DAY 6	DAY 7	DAY 8	DAY 9	DAY 10	
Soft-Boiled Eggs with Grape Tomatoes	Tomato and Zucchini Omelet	Blue Smoothie Bowl	Orange Creamsicle Smoothie	Chia Seed Pudding with Dried Apricots	**BREAKFAST**
Tomato and Watermelon Gazpacho Topped with Crab	Lemony Lentil Soup	Roasted Cauliflower and Squash Salad with Chicken	Cod and Summer Squash Pasta with Green Goddess Dressing	Smoked Salmon with Spring Salad	**LUNCH**
Cinnamon-Spiced Pumpkin Seeds	Fresh Blueberries	4 Black Sesame Seed Crackers	Miso Soup	Matcha Green Mylk	**SNACK**
Pan-Seared Steak with Cucumber Dill Salad	Treat Meal	Sautéed Cod over Ratatouille	Lamb Meatballs with Herbed Salad	Cauliflower Rice Bowl	**DINNER**
Peach Slices Dipped in 1 tablespoon Honey	2 Clementines	2 Fig and Coconut Balls	1 cup Watermelon Slices	Chocolate Almond Milk	**SNACK**

ETHEREAL'S MEAL PLAN

	DAY 1	DAY 2	DAY 3	DAY 4	DAY 5
BREAKFAST	Spiced Banana Coconut Smoothie	Sweet Strawberry Oatmeal Smoothie	Matcha Avocado Smoothie	Golden Smoothie Bowl	Chia Seed Pudding with Apricots and Macadamia Nuts
LUNCH	Mediterranean Salmon Salad	Smoked Trout and Vegetable Plate with Hemp and Chia Pesto	Shrimp and Veggie Avocado Bowl	Lemon Edamame and Avocado Rice Bowl	Seared Beef Skewers with Quinoa and Israeli Salad
SNACK	3 Sunflower Seed Crackers with Tahini	1 Superfood Bar	Cumin-Scented Chickpeas	Cacao, Coconut, and Goji Berry Trail Mix	Cacao-Infused Golden Mylk
DINNER	Pan-Seared Lemon Sole with Wild Arugula Salad	Halibut with Curried Vegetables and Potato	Seared Scallops over Sweet Pea Puree with Moroccan Carrot Salad	Hemp-Crusted Mahi Mahi with Roasted Vegetables	Cajun Fish Tacos with Summer Slaw
SNACK	24 Pistachios	1 cup Blackberries	8oz Kombucha	Two Dates with 4 Almonds	1 Coconut Macaroon

DAY 6	DAY 7	DAY 8	DAY 9	DAY 10	
Soft-Boiled Eggs with Grape Tomatoes with Gluten-Free Toast	Pan-Fried Eggs over Rice and Greens	Buckwheat Banana Pancakes	Vanilla and Pumpkin Seed Smoothie	Chia Seed Pudding with Dried Figs, Black Sesame Seeds, and Raw Honey	BREAKFAST
Soba Noodles with Scallions and Snap Peas	Beet Burger with Carrot Turmeric Hummus and BBQ 'Shrooms	Roasted Cauliflower and Squash Salad with Chicken	Cod with Summer Squash Pasta and a Green Goddess Dressing	Falafel over Greens and Purple Cabbage	LUNCH
Cinnamon-Spiced Pumpkin Seeds	Chocolate Chia Seed Pudding with Cacao Nibs	4 Black Sesame Seed Crackers with ¼ Avocado	Beet and Carrot Juice	Matcha Green Mylk	SNACK
Pan-Seared Steak with Cucumber Dill Salad	Treat Meal	Sautéed Cod over Ratatouille	Lamb Meatballs with Herbed Salad	Lemony Lentil Soup	DINNER
4 Fresh Figs	1 cup Blueberries	2 Fig and Coconut Balls	2 Cacao Matcha Truffles	2 Brazil Nuts Dipped in 2 teaspoons Tahini with Cinnamon	SNACK

CHAPTER 14

Recipes

===

Below are recipes for all of the dishes suggested on the archetype's meal plan. Unless otherwise specified, follow your archetype's suggested serving sizes for protein, fat, and carbs. You can also swap out different types of foods depending on your taste preferences and availability (for example, you can choose organic, grass-fed lamb instead of beef, or wild-caught organic cod instead of halibut) or add other vegetables corresponding to your archetype's chakra color for additional rebalancing. Just remember to always use organic, high-quality ingredients whenever possible.

BREAKFAST

As per the Food Fundamentals, your breakfast should be protein-based. Below are some of my favorite breakfast dishes, including smoothies, smoothie bowls, chia seed pudding, and eggs.

MORNING SMOOTHIE

ALL ARCHETYPES

Use this as the basic template for designing a smoothie perfect for your archetype. You can use any type of nondairy milk such as hemp, flax, almond, pea, or coconut, and add any of the fruits and vegetables recommended for your archetype, especially those associated with your archetype's chakra color. One caveat: only Ethereals or those eating for maintenance should include bananas. You can boost your smoothie with one or more superfoods, such as bee pollen, cacao, or unsweetened coconut flakes. If you are taking supplements in a powdered form, including the adrenal tonic, you can also add them to the smoothie.

SERVES 1

1 cup nut milk
1 cup fresh or frozen fruit
*2 tablespoons plant protein powder such as Beautifuel protein
    powder**
Handful of greens/vegetables, optional
1 teaspoon superfoods, optional

Place the nut milk, fruit, protein powder, greens, if using, and superfood, if using, in a blender and blend for 30 to 60 seconds until smooth.

*See Appendix C: Resources.

CHERRY CHOCOLATE SMOOTHIE

NURTURER

SERVES 1

1 cup almond milk

1 cup frozen cherries

2 tablespoons plant protein powder such as Beautifuel protein
powder

1 small red beet, peeled

1 teaspoon cacao

Place all of the ingredients in a blender and blend for 30 to 60 seconds until smooth. (If using a powerful blender, a raw beet can be used. If using a simple blender, add a cooked beet.)

STRAWBERRY HEMP SMOOTHIE

NURTURER

SERVES 1

1 cup hemp seed milk

1 cup frozen strawberries

2 tablespoons plant protein powder such as Beautifuel protein
powder

1 teaspoon hemp seeds, for garnish

Place the hemp milk, strawberries, and protein powder in a blender and blend for 30 to 60 seconds until smooth. Pour into a glass and top with hemp seeds.

PINEAPPLE GREEN SMOOTHIE

WONDER WOMAN

SERVES 1

1 cup almond milk

1 cup frozen pineapple

*2 tablespoons plant protein powder such as Beautifuel protein
   powder*

Handful of spinach

Handful of fresh mint, optional

Place the almond milk, pineapple, protein powder, spinach, and fresh mint, if
using, in the bowl of a blender and blend for 30 to 60 seconds until smooth.

GREEN DETOX SMOOTHIE

WONDER WOMAN

SERVES 1

1 cup hemp seed milk

$1/2$ cup frozen pineapple

$1/2$ pear, peeled

*2 tablespoons plant protein powder such as Beautifuel protein
   powder*

Handful of wild baby arugula

1 teaspoon bee pollen, for garnish

Place the hemp milk, pineapple, pear, protein powder, and arugula in a blender
and blend for 30 to 60 seconds until smooth. Pour into a glass and top with the
bee pollen.

KIWI SMOOTHIE

WONDER WOMAN

SERVES 1

1 cup almond milk

2 kiwifruit, peeled

2 tablespoons plant protein powder such as Beautifuel protein
   powder

Handful of kale

1 teaspoon bee pollen, for garnish

Place the almond milk, kiwi, protein powder, and kale in a blender and blend for 30 to 60 seconds until smooth. Pour into a glass and top with the bee pollen.

PAPAYA COCONUT SMOOTHIE

FEMME FATALE

SERVES 1

1 cup coconut milk

1 cup papaya

2 tablespoons plant protein powder such as Beautifuel protein
   powder

Handful of ice

1 teaspoon bee pollen, for garnish

Place the coconut milk, papaya, protein powder, and ice in a blender and blend for 30 to 60 seconds until smooth. Pour into a glass and top with the bee pollen.

GINGER MANGO SMOOTHIE

FEMME FATALE

SERVES 1

1 cup hemp seed milk

1 cup frozen mango

2 tablespoons plant protein powder such as Beautifuel protein powder

Pinch of ground ginger powder

1 teaspoon unsweetened coconut flakes, for garnish

Place the hemp milk, mango, protein powder, and ginger in a blender and blend for 30 to 60 seconds until smooth. Pour into a glass and top with coconut flakes.

MATCHA AVOCADO SMOOTHIE

ALL ARCHETYPES

SERVES 1

1 cup cashew milk

¼ avocado

2 tablespoons plant protein powder such as Beautifuel protein powder

½ teaspoon matcha powder

1 teaspoon raw honey

Pinch of ground cinnamon

Pinch of ground nutmeg

½ banana (Ethereal or maintenance only)

Place all of the ingredients in a blender and blend for 30 to 60 seconds until smooth.

ORANGE CREAMSICLE SMOOTHIE

FEMME FATALE

Created by Arielle Haspel from Be Well With Arielle

SERVES 1

1 cup coconut milk

1 orange, peeled

$^1\!/_2$ teaspoon ground ginger

$^1\!/_4$ teaspoon vanilla extract

1 date, pitted

2 tablespoons plant protein powder such as Beautifuel protein powder

$^1\!/_4$ avocado

Handful of ice (approximately 3 cubes)

Place all of the ingredients in a blender and blend for 30 to 60 seconds until smooth.

SCARLET RED SMOOTHIE

NURTURER

SERVES 1

1 cup cashew milk

$^1\!/_2$ cup raspberries

½ red apple, chopped

¼ red bell pepper, cored, seeded, chopped

2 tablespoons plant protein powder such as Beautifuel protein powder

1 teaspoon coconut oil

Place all of the ingredients in a blender and blend for 30 to 60 seconds until smooth.

SPICED BANANA COCONUT SMOOTHIE

ETHEREAL ONLY

SERVES 1

1 cup coconut milk

1 small banana

2 tablespoons plant protein powder such as Beautifuel protein powder

1 teaspoon coconut oil

1 teaspoon raw honey

Pinch of ground cinnamon

Pinch of ground nutmeg

Handful of ice

Place all of the ingredients in a blender and blend for 30 to 60 seconds until smooth.

SWEET STRAWBERRY OATMEAL SMOOTHIE

ETHEREAL ONLY

SERVES 1

1 cup almond milk

³/₄ cup frozen strawberries

¹/₂ cup gluten-free oats

1 tablespoon ground flaxseeds

2 tablespoons plant protein powder such as Beautifuel protein
   powder

1 teaspoon coconut oil

Place all of the ingredients in a blender and blend for 30 to 60 seconds until smooth.

VANILLA AND PUMPKIN SEED SMOOTHIE

ETHEREAL ONLY

SERVES 1

1 cup hemp seed milk

2 tablespoons pumpkin seeds

1 date, pitted

¹/₂ cup canned pumpkin, unsweetened

2 tablespoons plant protein powder such as Beautifuel protein
   powder

1 teaspoon coconut oil

Pinch of vanilla bean powder

Pinch of ground nutmeg

Place all of the ingredients in a blender and blend for 30 to 60 seconds until smooth.

GOLDEN SMOOTHIE BOWL

ALL ARCHETYPES

SERVES 1

$^3/_4$ cup unsweetened coconut milk

$^3/_4$ cup frozen mango ($^1/_2$ cup for Ethereal)

$^1/_2$ small banana (Ethereal only)

2 tablespoons plant protein powder such as Beautifuel protein powder

1 teaspoon coconut oil

$^1/_4$ teaspoon ground turmeric powder

Pinch of ground cinnamon

TO SERVE:

Pinch of freshly cracked black pepper

2 teaspoons unsweetened coconut flakes

1 teaspoon bee pollen

In the bowl of a blender, place the coconut milk, fruit, protein powder, coconut oil, turmeric, and cinnamon and blend for 30 to 60 seconds until smooth. If required, add more fruit or coconut milk to achieve the desired consistency. Pour into a bowl and top with pepper, coconut flakes, and bee pollen.

BLUE SMOOTHIE BOWL

WONDER WOMAN AND FEMME FATALE

SERVES 1

³/₄ cup cashew milk

¹/₂ pear, peeled

¹/₂ cup frozen wild blueberries

2 tablespoons plant protein powder such as Beautifuel protein
    powder

1 teaspoon coconut oil

¹/₂ teaspoon blue-green algae powder

TO SERVE:

10 blueberries

8 shelled crushed pistachios

In the bowl of a blender, place the cashew milk, pear, blueberries, protein powder, coconut oil, and algae powder and blend for 30 to 60 seconds until smooth. If required, add more fruit or coconut milk to achieve the desired consistency. Pour into a bowl and top with blueberries and pistachios.

PINK SMOOTHIE BOWL

NURTURER

SERVES 1

³/₄ cup coconut milk

1 cup strawberries

¹/₂ pink dragon fruit, peeled (optional)

2 tablespoons plant protein powder such as Beautifuel protein
  powder
1 teaspoon coconut oil

TO SERVE:

  1 tablespoon unsweetened coconut flakes
  1 tablespoon bee pollen

Place the coconut milk, strawberries, dragon fruit, if using, protein powder, and coconut oil in a food processor and blend for 30 to 60 seconds until smooth. If required, add more fruit or coconut milk to achieve the desired consistency. Pour into a bowl and top with coconut flakes and bee pollen.

CHIA SEED PUDDING

ALL ARCHETYPES

Chia seed pudding is not only highly nutrient-dense but also incredibly versatile. Serve this recipe with the toppings suggested on your archetype's meal plan or any other fruit, seeds, or nuts recommended for your archetype.

SERVES 1

  1 cup nut milk of your choice
  3 tablespoons chia seeds
  1 teaspoon raw honey, maple syrup, or coconut sugar
  Pinch of ground cinnamon

Combine all of the ingredients in a mason jar and shake until the seeds are immersed in the liquid. Let it sit for 15 minutes or overnight. If you'd like a warm version, heat the milk over medium heat before pouring over the chia seeds.

This will also reduce the time it takes for the seeds to soften, from 15 minutes down to 5 minutes.

CHIA SEED PUDDING WITH APRICOTS AND MACADAMIA NUTS

ETHEREAL ONLY (OTHER ARCHETYPES SEE ADJUSTMENTS BELOW)

SERVES 1

3 tablespoons chia seeds
1 cup coconut milk
1 teaspoon coconut sugar
Pinch of vanilla bean

TO SERVE:

4 dried apricots, chopped
6 macadamia nuts, chopped

Place the chia seeds, coconut milk, coconut sugar, and vanilla in a mason jar and shake vigorously. Let it sit for 15 minutes or overnight. When set, top with apricots and macadamia nuts.

FOR THE OTHER ARCHETYPES:

For Day 5, instead of the apricots and macadamia nuts, the Nurturer uses 3 tablespoons of raspberries, the Wonder Woman uses 1 golden kiwifruit, and the Femme Fatale uses 1 chopped peach.

For Day 10, Wonder Woman and Femme Fatale, skip the macadamia nuts. The Nurturer replaces the dried apricots with 2 fresh apricots. For Day 10 on the

Ethereal plan, replace the apricots and macadamia nuts with 2 dried figs and 1 tablespoon black sesame seeds. Replace the coconut sugar with 1 teaspoon raw honey.

BUCKWHEAT BANANA PANCAKES

ETHEREAL ONLY

SERVES 2

1 ¹/₄ cups almond milk
1 tablespoon freshly squeezed lemon juice
1 tablespoon coconut oil, melted and cooled, plus more for
    cooking
1 tablespoon maple syrup, plus more for serving
¹/₂ cup buckwheat flour
¹/₂ cup brown rice flour
1 teaspoon baking soda
¹/₂ teaspoon sea salt
1 banana, thinly sliced
Sprinkle of shredded unsweetened coconut
Handful of fresh or frozen blueberries

In a medium-sized bowl, whisk together the almond milk, lemon juice, coconut oil, and maple syrup. Add the buckwheat flour, brown rice flour, baking soda, salt, and banana and stir until combined. Heat a large skillet over medium heat and add a thin layer of coconut oil to the bottom of the pan. Pour the batter into the pan 1/4 cup at a time. Cook for about 1 minute until small bubbles form on the surface of the batter. Flip and cook for 1 minute more until the underside is golden brown. Serve with shredded coconut, blueberries, and maple syrup.

Leftover pancakes can be wrapped tightly and stored in the refrigerator for up to 2 days.

SOFT-BOILED EGGS WITH TOMATOES

ALL ARCHETYPES

SERVES 1

2 organic eggs
5 yellow or red grape tomatoes, sliced
Pink sea salt and cracked black pepper to taste
1 slice toasted gluten-free bread (Ethereal only)

Add 3 cups of water to a small saucepan. Place the whole eggs in the pan and bring the water to a boil over high heat. Boil for 6 minutes, then transfer the eggs to cold water. Peel the eggs, cut them in half, and place them on a plate with the tomatoes. Sprinkle the eggs and tomatoes with sea salt and cracked pepper. Serve with gluten-free toast if an Ethereal.

TOMATO AND ZUCCHINI OMELET

NURTURER, WONDER WOMAN, AND FEMME FATALE

SERVES 1

2 organic eggs
Pinch of sea salt
Pinch of freshly cracked black pepper
1 tablespoon coconut oil
1 small zucchini, cut into bite-size pieces

5 yellow or red grape tomatoes, sliced in half

Sprinkle of fresh parsley leaves

Crack the eggs into a small bowl. Add the salt, pepper, and a splash of water and beat. Heat an 8-inch pan over medium heat. Place the coconut oil in the pan and melt it to coat the bottom of the pan. Add the zucchini and tomatoes and sauté them until lightly browned and soft. Pour the egg mixture into the pan and swirl the pan to cover the vegetables with the egg. Cook for 2 minutes, until the egg is set and dry at the edges and slightly wet on top. Fold the omelet in half and slide off the pan onto a plate. Garnish with parsley.

PAN-FRIED EGGS OVER RICE AND GREENS

ETHEREAL ONLY

SERVES 1

2 tablespoons coconut oil

1/2 cup button mushrooms, sliced

Pinch of sea salt and freshly cracked black pepper

2 handfuls of greens (such as spinach, Swiss chard, or kale), torn into bite-size pieces

1/2 cup cooked brown rice, warmed

2 organic eggs

Pinch of fresh thyme leaves (optional)

Pinch of smoked paprika (optional)

In a small frying pan, heat 1 tablespoon of coconut oil over medium heat. Add the mushrooms and cook until golden and soft. Sprinkle with a pinch of salt. Add the greens and sauté until wilted. Place the brown rice on a plate and top with the cooked vegetables. In the same pan, heat the remaining tablespoon of coconut oil over medium-high heat. When warm, break the eggs into the pan and cook until the edges are crispy and the white is set. If you prefer your eggs fully cooked, reduce the heat to medium and cover the pan until the yolks are cooked all the way through. Season with salt and pepper. Slide the eggs on top of the rice and vegetables. Top with thyme and smoked paprika, if desired.

LUNCH

MEDITERRANEAN SALMON SALAD

WONDER WOMAN, FEMME FATALE, AND ETHEREAL

SERVES 1

1 tablespoon pine nuts

$1/2$ small head of Bibb lettuce

2 sprigs of fresh mint

4 radishes, cut into quarters

$1/2$ yellow bell pepper, cored, seeded, and sliced (Femme Fatale,
   replace with orange bell pepper)

$1/4$ cup canned cannellini beans, rinsed (Femme Fatale, replace
   beans with $1/4$ cup cooked yellow squash; Ethereal, increase to
   $1/2$ cup)

1 tablespoon Lemon Vinaigrette (page 210)

1 tablespoon coconut oil

4 ounces wild salmon

In a small frying pan, toast the pine nuts over low heat for about 2 minutes. While the pine nuts are toasting, separate the leaves of the Bibb lettuce onto a plate. Top with the mint, radishes, bell pepper, and white beans. When the pine nuts are toasted, add to the salad and drizzle the salad with the vinaigrette.

In a small frying pan, melt the coconut oil over medium heat. Add the salmon to the pan, skin-side down, and cook for 4 minutes or until cooked halfway through. Flip the salmon and cook for 2 to 4 minutes more, depending on how well you like your salmon cooked. Serve on top of the salad.

PAN-ROASTED WILD SALMON WITH BEET AND SPINACH SALAD

NURTURER

SERVES 1

1 tablespoon coconut oil
One 5-ounce wild salmon fillet
Sea salt and freshly cracked pepper to taste
$^1/_4$ lemon
4 handfuls of baby spinach
$^1/_2$ small raw beet, peeled and grated
2 carrots, peeled and grated
1 tablespoon Green Goddess Dressing (page 211)
*1 tablespoon toasted hazelnuts, chopped**

Melt the coconut oil in a small skillet over medium heat. Add the salmon, skin-side down, and cook for 4 minutes or until the fish is cooked about halfway through. Flip the salmon and cook for 2 to 4 minutes more, depending on how well you like your salmon cooked. Transfer the salmon to a plate, season to taste with salt and pepper, and let it rest while you make the salad.

Place the spinach, beets, and carrots in a large bowl. Drizzle with the dressing and toss to coat. Mound the salad on the plate next to the fish and sprinkle with toasted hazelnuts.

*To toast hazelnuts, place the hazelnuts in a small skillet over medium heat and cook for 1 to 2 minutes. Stir, using a wooden spoon, to ensure that they don't stick to the pan. The hazelnuts are toasted when they give off a rich, nutty aroma.

SMOKED TROUT AND VEGETABLE PLATE WITH HEMP AND CHIA PESTO

ALL ARCHETYPES

Pesto created by natural food chef Mikaela Reuben

SERVES 8

HEMP AND CHIA PESTO

> 1 $^1/_2$ teaspoons chia seeds
>
> 2 cups packed fresh basil
>
> $^2/_3$ cup hemp hearts
>
> 1 $^1/_4$ teaspoons garlic, minced
>
> $^1/_2$ teaspoon sea salt
>
> 2 tablespoons freshly squeezed lemon juice
>
> 1 tablespoon nutritional yeast
>
> 1 $^1/_2$ teaspoons tamari

SMOKED TROUT AND VEGETABLE PLATE

> 3 cups assorted steamed or raw vegetables, such as yellow tomatoes, heirloom carrots, cauliflower, beets, asparagus, endive leaves, or radishes
>
> $^1/_4$ cup cooked chickpeas, rinsed (Nurturer, replace with $^1/_2$ cup broccoli florets; Ethereal, increase to $^1/_2$ cup)
>
> 4 ounces smoked trout (Nurturer, increase to 5 ounces)

Make the pesto: Place the chia seeds in a bowl with 2 tablespoons water and set aside for 15 minutes. Pour the soaked chia seeds into the bowl of a blender or food processor and add the basil, hemp hearts, garlic, salt, lemon juice, nutritional yeast, and tamari. Blend until creamy, stopping once or twice to scrape down the sides of the bowl. Taste and add more salt, tamari, or lemon juice if desired.

Arrange the vegetables, chickpeas, and fish on a plate with a small bowl of the pesto for dipping the veggies.

SHRIMP AND VEGGIE AVOCADO BOWL

ALL ARCHETYPES

SERVES 1

1 tablespoon coconut oil

³/₄ cup mushrooms, cleaned

Pinch of sea salt and cracked black pepper to taste

4 cups assorted greens, such as spinach, kale, asparagus, and green beans

1 tablespoon extra virgin olive oil

¹/₄ cup cooked quinoa (Nurturer, skip; Ethereal, increase to ¹/₂ cup)

4 ounces cooked shrimp (Nurturer, increase to 5 ounces)

¹/₄ avocado, sliced

Juice of ¹/₂ lemon

1 teaspoon grated lemon zest

In a frying pan, melt the coconut oil over medium heat. Add the mushrooms and the salt and pepper to taste. Cook the mushrooms thoroughly, flipping them occasionally. Add water if the mushrooms start to stick to the pan. When the mushrooms are soft, transfer them to a plate. In the same pan, add 1/2 cup water and bring it to a boil. Add the greens and cover them with a lid. If using spinach or another tender green, add it to the pan after the other vegetables have almost finished cooking. Once the vegetables are tender, drain the water from the pan. Add the olive oil and cook for 1 minute more. Add salt to taste.

To serve, place the cooked greens, warmed mushrooms, and quinoa, if using, in a small bowl. Top with the shrimp and sliced avocado. Squeeze lemon juice over the dish and sprinkle with the lemon zest.

NOTE Shrimp can be warmed by gently heating it in a frying pan for 2 minutes.

TURKEY (OR SALMON) BURGER WITH SALSA

NURTURER, WONDER WOMAN, AND FEMME FATALE

SERVES 1

*4 ounces organic ground turkey (Nurturer, replace with 5 ounces
   wild salmon*)*
1 teaspoon Dijon mustard
1 small shallot, peeled and grated
Sea salt and freshly cracked black pepper
1 tablespoon extra virgin olive oil
3 handfuls of baby lettuce
1 small Persian cucumber, chopped
10 sugar snap peas
6 fresh mint leaves, torn
*$1/4$ cup cooked black rice (Nurturer, skip; Ethereal, increase to $1/2$
   cup)*

1 tablespoon Lemon Vinaigrette (page 210)
1 tablespoon salsa, such as Whole Foods organic salsa
¼ avocado

Place the turkey, mustard, and shallot in a medium-sized bowl. Season with a large pinch of salt and a few grinds of pepper. Mix with your hands until just combined. Shape the mixture into a patty. Heat the olive oil in a medium-sized pan over medium-high heat. When hot, add the patty to the pan and cook for about 5 minutes on each side, or until the desired doneness. While the patty is cooking, place the lettuce, cucumber, sugar snap peas, mint, and rice in a small serving bowl and toss with the dressing.

Once the patty is finished cooking, place it on a small plate and top with the salsa and avocado.

*If using salmon instead of turkey, cut it into 1-inch cubes, place the salmon pieces in the bowl of a food processor or blender, add the mustard and shallot, and blend until still chunky. Continue with the rest of the directions, decreasing the cook time to 3 minutes on each side.

TURMERIC CHICKEN (OR SEARED BEEF SKEWERS) WITH QUINOA AND ISRAELI SALAD

ALL ARCHETYPES

SERVES 1

Leaves from 1 sprig of fresh oregano
½ teaspoon ground turmeric powder
2 tablespoons olive oil
Sea salt and freshly cracked black pepper

One 4-ounce boneless organic chicken breast (Nurturer, increase to 5 ounces; Ethereal, replace with organic, grass-fed beef, sliced)

¼ cup cooked quinoa (Nurturer, replace with 2 tablespoons hemp seeds; Ethereal, increase to ½ cup)

1 Persian cucumber, chopped

1 heirloom tomato, seeded and cut into bite-size pieces

1 scallion, sliced

¼ cup fresh parsley, chopped

2 tablespoons fresh mint leaves, chopped

1 tablespoon Lemon Vinaigrette (page 210)

Combine the oregano, turmeric, olive oil, and salt in a large bowl. Add the chicken breast and toss to coat.* Set aside while you make the salad.

In a small serving bowl, mix the quinoa (or hemp seeds), cucumber, tomato, scallion, parsley, and mint together. Toss the salad with the dressing.

Heat a medium pan over medium-high heat. When hot, take the chicken out of the marinade and cook for about 4 minutes on each side, or until cooked through. Once cooked, add the chicken (or beef skewers) to the salad and serve.

*If using beef instead of chicken, add the slices to three skewers (soak the skewers in water before using so they don't burn). Brush with olive oil and sprinkle with salt and pepper. Turn oven on to broil and broil for 3 minutes on each side.

LEMONY LENTIL SOUP

WONDER WOMAN, FEMME FATALE, AND ETHEREAL

Created by Robyn Youkilis, author of Go with Your Gut

SERVES 4

3 tablespoons extra-virgin olive oil, plus more for drizzling

1 large onion, chopped

2 garlic cloves, minced

1 tablespoon tomato paste

1 teaspoon ground cumin

1/2 teaspoon sea salt

1/4 teaspoon freshly cracked black pepper

Pinch of ground chili or cayenne powder

1 quart organic vegetable, chicken, or bone broth

1 cup red lentils

1 large carrot, diced

Juice of 1 lemon

3 tablespoons chopped fresh parsley

TO SERVE:

Sprinkling of chopped herbs such as parsley and cilantro

3 Sunflower-Seed Crackers (page 221) (Ethereal only)

In a large pot, heat the olive oil over medium-low heat. Add the onion and garlic and sauté for 4 to 6 minutes, until they are golden. Stir in the tomato paste, cumin, salt, pepper, and chili powder and sauté for 2 minutes.

Add the broth, 2 cups of water, the lentils, and the carrot. Bring to a simmer, then partially cover the pot and raise the heat to medium-low. Simmer until the lentils are soft, about 30 minutes. Taste and add more salt if necessary.

Place half of the soup in the bowl of a blender and puree it. Add it back to the pot. Stir in the lemon juice and parsley. Pour a quarter of the soup into a bowl and top with a sprinkle of fresh herbs. An Ethereal can serve the soup with sunflower-seed crackers.

CHICKEN AND VEGETABLE SOUP

NURTURER

SERVES 2

1 quart organic chicken stock

1 small onion, diced

2 stalks celery, chopped

4 carrots, peeled and cut into bite-size pieces

1 bay leaf

1 teaspoon sea salt

4 handfuls of greens (such as spinach, kale, or Swiss chard), torn
  into bite-size pieces

10 ounces roasted organic chicken breast, shredded

Chives, chopped

Cracked black pepper to taste

In a large pot, bring the chicken stock to a boil over medium-high heat. Add the onion, celery, carrots, bay leaf, and salt and reduce the heat to medium-low. Simmer until the vegetables are soft, about 10 minutes. Add the greens and shredded chicken. Cook until the greens wilt and the chicken is warmed through. Discard the bay leaf. Ladle into two bowls and top with chives and black pepper.

Extra soup can be stored in the refrigerator for up to 2 days.

TOMATO AND WATERMELON
GAZPACHO TOPPED WITH CRAB

NURTURER, WONDER WOMAN, AND FEMME FATALE

SERVES 2

2 beefsteak or heirloom tomatoes, chopped

2 cups watermelon, cubed

$\frac{1}{2}$ cucumber, peeled and diced

1 orange bell pepper, cored, seeded, and diced

1 scallion, sliced

1 garlic clove, peeled

4 sprigs of fresh mint

$\frac{1}{4}$ cup fresh basil leaves

Sea salt and freshly cracked black pepper to taste

Pinch of cayenne pepper

$\frac{1}{2}$ avocado, cubed

10 grape tomatoes, sliced in half

8 ounces cooked crab meat (Nurturer, increase to 10 ounces)

8 flax crackers, such as Doctor in the Kitchen Flackers

Place the chopped tomatoes, watermelon, cucumber, bell pepper, scallion, garlic, mint, and basil in a medium-sized bowl and toss together. In batches, add the mixture to the bowl of a high-speed blender and blend for 60 seconds until smooth. Season with salt, black pepper, and cayenne. Pour the gazpacho into two bowls and top with avocado, grape tomatoes, and crab meat. Serve with the crackers on the side.

ROASTED CAULIFLOWER AND SQUASH SALAD WITH CHICKEN

ALL ARCHETYPES

Created by Amie Valpone from The Healthy Apple

SERVES 1

1/4 head cauliflower, cut into 1/2-inch florets

1/4 cup delicata squash, seeded and cut into 1/2-inch slices
   (Nurturer, skip. Ethereal, increase to 1/2 cup)

2 carrots, peeled and sliced into matchsticks

1 tablespoon olive oil

Sea salt and freshly cracked black pepper to taste

2 cups wild arugula

1/2 cup thinly sliced red cabbage

1 medium heirloom tomato, diced

1/2 yellow bell pepper, cored, seeded, and sliced (Nurturer,
   substitute red bell pepper; Femme Fatale, substitute orange
   bell pepper)

1/2 small English cucumber, diced

4 ounces organic rotisserie chicken (Nurturer, increase to 5 ounces)

1 tablespoon Tahini Dressing (page 211)

1 tablespoon hemp seeds

Preheat the oven to 375°F. Line a baking pan with parchment paper. Mound the cauliflower, squash, if using, and carrots on the baking sheet, drizzle with the olive oil, and toss to coat. Spread into a single layer and season with salt and black pepper. Roast for 30 minutes or until golden brown and tender. Transfer to a large bowl and set aside to cool. Add the arugula, cabbage, tomato, bell pepper, and cucumber. Shred the chicken and add to the salad.

Drizzle with the dressing and toss gently to coat. Season with salt and black pepper to taste. Garnish with the hemp seeds and serve immediately.

COD AND SUMMER SQUASH PASTA WITH GREEN GODDESS DRESSING

ALL ARCHETYPES

SERVES 1

2 medium summer squash

1 tablespoon olive oil (optional)

Sea salt and freshly cracked black pepper

2 tablespoons Green Goddess Dressing (page 211)

One 4-ounce cod fillet, cooked (Nurturer, increase to 5 ounces)

$1/2$ cup cooked butternut squash, diced (Ethereal only)

Small handful of fresh cilantro leaves

$1/2$ teaspoon lemon zest

Use a mandoline or knife to cut the squash into thin, noodle-like strips. You may leave the noodles raw or sauté them in a small pan with the olive oil until slightly soft. Transfer the noodles to a medium-sized bowl and add the dressing. Add the butternut squash, if using. Pull the cooked cod apart so that it is in bite-size pieces and toss with the noodles. Top with the cilantro and lemon zest and serve.

SMOKED SALMON WITH KALE AND FENNEL SALAD

NURTURER

SERVES 1

$1/2$ bunch of kale

1 tablespoon Lemon Vinaigrette (page 210)

Pinch of sea salt

$1/4$ small red onion, diced

$1/4$ small fennel bulb, shaved

$1/4$ cup fresh parsley leaves

5 ounces smoked 8 hazelnuts wild salmon

Remove the kale leaves from their stems and discard the stems. Place the leaves on top of one another and roll them up like a burrito. Slice them width-wise into thin ribbons. Place the kale in a medium-sized bowl and massage it with the dressing and salt until the kale softens. Add the red onion, fennel, parsley, and hazelnuts and toss together. Serve the salad with the salmon.

SMOKED SALMON WITH SPRING SALAD

WONDER WOMAN AND FEMME FATALE

SERVES 1

2 cups spinach

1 cup mixed greens

2 radishes, cut into quarters

$1/2$ yellow or orange bell pepper, cored, seeded, and sliced

$1/4$ cup cooked asparagus, trimmed and sliced into bite-size pieces

$1/4$ cup fresh parsley leaves

2 small new potatoes, cooked and sliced

1 tablespoon pumpkin seeds

1 tablespoon Green Goddess Dressing (page 211)

4 ounces smoked wild salmon

In a large bowl, toss the spinach, greens, radishes, bell pepper, asparagus, parsley, new potatoes, and pumpkin seeds with the dressing. Transfer the mixture to a serving plate and top with the salmon.

LEMON, EDAMAME, AND AVOCADO RICE BOWL WITH CHICKEN

ETHEREAL ONLY

Created by natural food chef Candice Kumai

SERVES 1

1 tablespoon Lemon Tamari Dressing (below)

½ cup cooked brown rice

½ cup shelled edamame

2 cups wild baby arugula

4 ounces cooked organic chicken breast, thinly sliced

¼ avocado, thinly sliced

Place the dressing and rice in a medium-sized bowl and toss to coat. Add the edamame and arugula and toss gently to combine. Transfer to a serving bowl and top with the chicken and avocado.

LEMON TAMARI DRESSING

MAKES 2 SERVINGS

2 tablespoon tamari

1 tablespoon toasted sesame oil

Juice of 1 lemon

1 teaspoon dried oregano

1 teaspoon finely grated lemon zest (optional)

In a large bowl, whisk together the tamari, sesame oil, lemon juice, oregano, and lemon zest, if using, until well combined.

SOBA NOODLES WITH SCALLIONS AND SNAP PEAS

ETHEREAL ONLY

SERVES 1

2 tablespoons coconut oil

1 handful button mushrooms, chopped into bite-size pieces

1 scallion, chopped

1 cup sugar snap peas

Sea salt and freshly cracked black pepper

4 ounces extra-firm tofu, sliced into $1/2$-inch pieces

$1/2$ cup cooked soba noodles

3 cups spinach

$1/4$ cup fresh cilantro, chopped

$1/4$ avocado, sliced

1 teaspoon lemon zest

Sea salt and cracked black pepper

Heat a large pan over medium heat. Add 1 tablespoon coconut oil and swirl until it's melted and coats the pan. Add the mushrooms and scallion to the pan and cook for about 5 minutes, until golden. Add the sugar snap peas and a pinch of salt. Cook for about 3 minutes or until the peas are soft but still green.

Meanwhile, add the remaining 1 tablespoon of coconut oil to a medium frying pan over medium heat. Once hot, add the tofu slices and cook for about 3 minutes on each side, until brown.

While the tofu is cooking, add the cooked noodles, spinach, and cilantro to the pan with the mushrooms and sugar snap peas. Stir until everything is combined and the spinach wilts.

Transfer the soba noodles and vegetables to a plate and add the tofu. Top with the avocado, lemon zest, and salt and pepper to taste.

BEET BURGER WITH CARROT TURMERIC HUMMUS AND BBQ 'SHROOMS

ETHEREAL ONLY

Created by Elenore Bendel Zahn, founder of Earthsprout

SERVES 4

3 tablespoons coconut oil, plus more as needed
1 cup button mushrooms, cleaned and thinly sliced
2 small beets, scrubbed
2 15-ounce cans black beans, drained and rinsed
$\frac{1}{2}$ cup chickpea flour
1 tablespoon coriander seeds
1 teaspoon caraway seeds
$\frac{1}{2}$ teaspoon freshly cracked black pepper
$\frac{1}{4}$ teaspoon sea salt
2 garlic cloves, minced
Handful of baby greens
2 tablespoons Carrot Turmeric Hummus (page 216)
$\frac{1}{4}$ cup BBQ 'Shrooms (recipe below)

Heat 1 tablespoon of the coconut oil in a medium cast-iron skillet. Once hot, add the mushrooms. Cook for about 5 minutes, until golden brown on all sides while stirring as little as possible. The mushrooms should be as dry as possible.

Place the mushrooms in the bowl of a food processor and add the beets, black beans, chickpea flour, coriander seeds, caraway seeds, pepper, salt, and garlic. Pulse the ingredients until it forms a sticky mixture and let it rest for at least 15 minutes (to let the chickpea flour work its magic) or overnight if you want to prep in advance.

Form the mixture into small patties using 1/4 cup of the mixture per patty. Heat another tablespoon of coconut oil in a medium-sized pan over medium heat. Once the oil is sizzling, fry the beet patties until golden on both sides. Add fresh oil for the next batch and continue frying until all of the patties are done.

To serve, place two burgers on a handful of baby greens and top with carrot hummus and BBQ 'Shrooms. Leftovers can be stored in an airtight container in the fridge for up to 1 week.

BBQ 'SHROOMS

2 large handfuls of oyster mushrooms (about 2/3 cup)

1/4 teaspoon sea salt

1/2 teaspoon tomato puree

1 teaspoon dark miso

1/2 teaspoon liquid smoke

1 garlic clove, minced

1/2 teaspoon coconut oil

Slice the mushrooms into thin strips and place them in a dry pan over medium heat. Add the salt and fry the mushrooms for about 5 minutes, until they are golden and dry, stirring as little as possible. Meanwhile, in a small bowl, whisk together the tomato puree, miso, liquid smoke, garlic, 1/2 teaspoon water, and the coconut oil. Add the mixture to the pan of mushrooms. Toss to cover and fry for 1 minute more. Serve immediately. Store leftovers in an airtight container in the fridge for up to 1 week.

FALAFEL OVER GREENS AND PURPLE CABBAGE

Created by McKel Hill from Nutrition Stripped

SERVES 2

1/4 cup raw sunflower seeds, shelled

1 cup cooked peas

3 tablespoons red onion, chopped

1 tablespoon fresh parsley, chopped

1 tablespoon fresh cilantro, chopped

1 tablespoon fresh mint, chopped

1 garlic clove, minced

1 tablespoon olive oil

1 tablespoon tahini

Juice of 1/2 lemon (about 2 tablespoons)

1 1/2 teaspoons brown rice flour

1/2 teaspoon baking powder

1/2 teaspoon chili powder

1/2 teaspoon ground cumin

1/2 teaspoon sea salt

Freshly cracked black pepper

4 cups steamed or sautéed greens (kale, spinach, or Swiss chard)
  and cabbage

Preheat the oven to 375° F. Place the sunflower seeds in the bowl of a blender or a food processor and pulse for 30 seconds or until coarsely chopped. Add the peas and pulse for 1 minute, pausing to scrape down the sides of the bowl. Keep pulsing until the mixture is slightly coarse and well combined. Transfer the mixture to a medium-sized bowl and add the onion, parsley, cilantro, mint, garlic, olive oil, tahini, lemon juice, brown rice flour, baking powder, chili powder, cumin, salt, and pepper. Stir the mixture until combined into a "dough."

Using your hands, form 18 small falafel balls and place them on a baking pan. Bake for 25 to 30 minutes, turning each falafel halfway through the baking process until all are evenly golden brown. To serve, place the steamed or sautéed greens and cabbage on a plate and top with 3 falafel.

Store the extra falafel in an airtight glass container for up to 1 week. Reheat by popping them into the oven or toaster oven until heated through and crisp.

DINNER

PAN-SEARED LEMON SOLE WITH WILD ARUGULA SALAD

ALL ARCHETYPES

SERVES 1

$1/4$ cup sweet potatoes, sliced into $1/4$-inch rounds (Nurturer, omit;
Ethereal, increase to $1/2$ cup)
1 tablespoon coconut oil
Pinch of sea salt
1 tablespoon pine nuts
2 handfuls of wild baby arugula
1 handful of shredded kale
$1/4$ small fennel bulb, shaved
1 small Persian cucumber, chopped
1 tablespoon Lemon Vinaigrette (page 210)
1 tablespoon olive oil

One 4-ounce lemon sole fillet (Nurturer, increase to 5 ounces)
Freshly cracked black pepper
Zest and juice of ½ lemon
Fresh herbs, such as parsley, chives, and dill, optional

Preheat the oven to 400°F. Coat both sides of the sweet potato slices, if using, with the coconut oil and place them on a baking pan in one layer. Sprinkle with salt. Bake for 10 minutes, then flip the rounds over and bake for 10 minutes more. Once the sweet potatoes are crispy on both sides, remove from the oven.

While the sweet potatoes are cooking, toast the pine nuts in a cast-iron skillet over medium heat, stirring with a wooden spoon to stop them from sticking and burning, about 3 minutes. Once lightly toasted, add them to a medium bowl along with the arugula, kale, fennel, and cucumber and toss with the dressing.

Heat the olive oil in a medium-sized pan over medium heat. When the oil is warm, add the lemon sole fillet. Season with salt and pepper and cook for 3 minutes. Flip and season the other side. Cook for 2 to 3 minutes more or until the fish is the same color throughout and flakes easily.

Transfer the fish to a plate. Sprinkle the lemon zest and lemon juice over the fish and season with salt. Serve with the salad and roasted sweet potatoes.

HALIBUT WITH CURRIED VEGETABLES AND POTATO

ALL ARCHETYPES

SERVES 2

1 tablespoon coconut oil

1 small onion, diced

2 garlic cloves, chopped

2 teaspoons fresh ginger, minced

$\frac{1}{2}$ cup new potatoes, diced small (Nurturer, omit; Ethereal,
   increase to 1 cup)

Sea salt to taste

1 yellow bell pepper, cored, seeded, and sliced

1 zucchini, sliced

2 cups cauliflower florets

1 large beefsteak tomato, chopped

1 teaspoon ground turmeric powder

2 teaspoons ground coriander

2 teaspoons ground cumin

Two 4-ounce halibut fillets, cut into 2-inch cubes (Nurturer,
   increase to 5 ounces)

Juice of 1 lemon

$\frac{1}{4}$ cup fresh cilantro leaves, chopped

Melt the coconut oil in a large saucepan over medium heat. Add the onion, garlic, ginger, potatoes, if using, and a pinch of salt. Cook, stirring frequently, for about 5 minutes, until the vegetables soften. Add the bell pepper, zucchini, cauliflower, tomato, turmeric, coriander, and cumin and stir to coat the vegetables with the spices. Add $\frac{1}{4}$ cup water if the tomato is not juicy. Cover the saucepan and simmer for 5 minutes. Add the halibut and cook for 5 minutes more, or until the fish is opaque throughout. Stir in the lemon juice, salt to taste, and cilantro, then serve.

SEARED SCALLOPS OVER SWEET PEA (OR CAULIFLOWER) PUREE WITH MOROCCAN CARROT SALAD

ALL ARCHETYPES

SERVES 1

CARROT SALAD

3 medium carrots

2 dates, pitted and chopped

1 tablespoon shelled pistachios, chopped

DRESSING

1 tablespoon extra-virgin olive oil

Juice of ½ navel orange

Pinch of ground cinnamon

Pinch of ground cumin

Pinch of sea salt

Dash of raw honey

1 garlic clove, smashed

PEA OR CAULIFLOWER PUREE

1 cup frozen sweet peas (Nurturer, substitute 1 cup cooked
cauliflower, chopped, to increase cruciferous vegetable intake)

1 tablespoon fresh mint leaves, chopped

1 lemon

Sea salt and freshly cracked black pepper
to taste

SCALLOPS

2 tablespoons olive oil

Sea salt and freshly cracked black pepper

4 scallops (Nurturer, increase to 5)

1/2 cup cooked purple potatoes (Ethereal only)

Make the carrot salad: Peel the carrots, then use the peeler to shave the carrots into thin ribbons. Place the ribbons in a large bowl with the dates and pistachios.

Make the dressing: Combine all of the dressing ingredients in a mason jar and shake vigorously. Drizzle over the salad and toss to coat.

Make the puree: Cook the frozen peas according to the directions on the package. Once cooked, place them (or the cauliflower) in the bowl of a blender and add the mint, a squeeze of lemon juice, and a touch of water. Blend until the mixture is smooth. Season with a pinch of salt and pepper. (I recommend doubling this recipe and using the leftover puree as a dip for a snack with crudités.)

Prepare the scallops: Heat the olive oil in a sauté pan over high heat. When the oil starts to sizzle, salt and pepper the scallops and add them to the pan, making sure they do not touch each other. Sear for 1 to 2 minutes on each side until a golden crust forms. Serve immediately on top of the pea or cauliflower puree with carrot salad and potatoes, if using, on the side. Drizzle with leftover dressing, as desired.

HEMP-CRUSTED MAHI MAHI
WITH ROASTED VEGETABLES

ALL ARCHETYPES

SERVES 2

1/2 cup baby potatoes, diced (Nurturer, omit; Ethereal, increase to
   1 cup)

2 small carrots, cut into bite-size pieces

½ yellow bell pepper, cored, seeded, and sliced (Nurturer,
    substitute red bell pepper)
1 large fennel bulb, cut into bite-size pieces
2 cups cauliflower, chopped
2 tablespoons extra-virgin olive oil, plus more for drizzling
Sea salt and freshly cracked black pepper to taste
¼ lemon, thinly sliced
2 fresh rosemary sprigs
2 fresh oregano sprigs
Two 4-ounce mahi mahi fillets (Nurturer, increase to 5 ounces)
1 tablespoon hemp seeds
Pinch of dried red pepper flakes
Handful of micro greens

Preheat the oven to 375°F. Put the baby potatoes, carrots, bell pepper, fennel, and cauliflower in a medium-sized bowl. Add the olive oil and a pinch of salt and black pepper. Toss to coat. Place the vegetables on a baking pan and roast for 10 minutes. Shake the pan so the vegetables don't stick and bake for 10 minutes more, or until the vegetables are golden on the outside but can be pierced easily with a fork. Add more salt and black pepper in the last 5 minutes to the vegetables.

While the vegetables are roasting, line a second baking pan with parchment paper and drizzle olive oil on it. Top with the lemon slices and half of the rosemary and oregano. Season the mahi mahi on both sides with salt, black pepper, hemp seeds, and red pepper flakes before placing it on top of the lemon slices and herbs. Cover with aluminum foil. Bake for 15 minutes, until the fish is flaky. Open the aluminum foil to allow the hemp seeds to form a crust and roast for another 5 minutes. Serve with the roasted vegetables and micro greens.

CAJUN FISH TACOS WITH SUMMER SLAW

ALL ARCHETYPES

SERVES 1

DRESSING

> 1¹/₂ teaspoons lemon juice
>
> Dash of raw honey
>
> Sea salt and freshly cracked black pepper
>
> 1 tablespoon extra-virgin olive oil

SUMMER SLAW

> ¹/₂ cup red cabbage, thinly sliced
>
> ¹/₂ cup green cabbage, thinly sliced
>
> 2 carrots, peeled and grated
>
> ¹/₄ avocado, diced
>
> ¹/₄ cup fresh cilantro

FISH TACO

> One 4-ounce striped bass, mahi mahi, or whitefish fillet (Nurturer,
>   increase to 5 ounces)
>
> Pinch sea salt and freshly cracked black pepper
>
> 1 tablespoon Cajun spices
>
> 1 tablespoon of extra-virgin olive oil
>
> 1 medium-size corn tortilla (Nurturer, omit; Ethereal, increase to 2
>   tortillas)

Make the dressing: Whisk together the lemon juice, honey, salt, and pepper. While whisking, add the olive oil until fully combined.

Make the summer slaw: In a separate medium-sized bowl, add the cabbage, carrots, avocado, and cilantro. Pour in the dressing and toss to coat. Let the slaw sit while you cook the fish.

Make the fish taco: Pat the fish dry and season on both sides with salt, pepper, and Cajun spices. Heat the olive oil in a pan over medium heat. When warm, add the fish and cook for 2 minutes. Flip the fish and cook until the fish is the same color throughout and flakes easily.

Lightly toast the corn tortilla over an open flame or warm in a cast-iron pan over low heat.

To serve, add half of the fish to the corn tortilla and top with summer slaw. Serve the remainder of the fish on the plate with rest of the slaw. Ethereal can add the remaining slaw to the second tortilla.

SAUTÉED COD OVER RATATOUILLE

ALL ARCHETYPES

SERVES 2

RATATOUILLE

2 tablespoons olive oil

$1/2$ small onion, diced

1 garlic clove, minced

1 medium eggplant, peeled and cut into $1/2$-inch pieces
    (about $1^1/2$ cups)

Sea salt

2 small zucchinis, cut into bite-size pieces

1 red bell pepper, cored, seeded, and sliced

One 15-ounce can diced tomatoes

$1/4$ teaspoon dried oregano, crumbled

¹/₄ teaspoon dried thyme, crumbled

Freshly cracked black pepper

COD

2 tablespoons olive oil

Two 4-ounce cod fillets (Nurturer, increase to 5 ounces)

Sea salt and freshly cracked black pepper

1 cup cooked brown rice (Ethereal only)

Make the ratatouille: In a large pan, heat the olive oil over medium-low heat. Add the onion and garlic and cook for 3 minutes, or until soft. Add the eggplant and a pinch of salt. Cook, stirring occasionally, until the eggplant has softened. Stir in the zucchini and bell pepper. When the vegetables are tender, add the tomatoes and cook for 5 minutes. Add the oregano and thyme and season with salt and black pepper to taste. Keep warm while preparing the fish.

Make the fish: Heat the olive oil in a medium-sized pan over medium heat. Season the cod with salt and black pepper. When the pan is warm, add the cod fillets and cook for 3 minutes on each side, until the fish is the same color throughout and flakes easily. Transfer the fish to a plate and serve over the warmed ratatouille and rice, if using.

PAN-SEARED STEAK (OR GRILLED SHRIMP) WITH CUCUMBER DILL SALAD

ALL ARCHETYPES

SERVES 1

CUCUMBER DILL SALAD

1 tablespoon olive oil

¹/₄ cup baby potatoes, cut into bite-size pieces (Nurturer, omit)

Pinch of sea salt

1 Persian cucumber, diced

½ cup cherry tomatoes, cut in half

2 tablespoons parsley

1 tablespoon dill, chopped

Juice of ½ lemon

STEAK (OR SHRIMP)

4 ounces grass-fed steak (Nurturer, replace with 5 ounces cooked shrimp)

Cracked black pepper

Kosher salt

1 tablespoon coconut oil

Make the salad: In a medium frying pan, heat the olive oil over medium heat. Add the potatoes and cook for 10 minutes, stirring frequently, until tender. If the edges are getting crispy before the inside is cooked, reduce the temperature. Season with salt. Place the potatoes in a medium-sized bowl and add the cucumber, tomatoes, parsley, dill, and lemon juice before transferring to a salad plate.

Make the steak: Cover the steak with cracked pepper and salt to prevent the steak from sticking to the pan. Place the coconut oil in a cast-iron skillet over medium-high heat. When the oil is hot, add the steak and sear for 3 minutes on each side. Transfer the steak to a plate and cover with aluminum foil and allow it to rest for 3 minutes, so the meat can continue to cook. Increase the cooking time if the desired doneness is greater than medium. If using shrimp, warm, if desired.

Serve the steak (or shrimp) with the salad.

LAMB (OR TURKEY) MEATBALLS WITH HERBED SALAD

ALL ARCHETYPES

SERVES 2

TOMATO SAUCE

> 1 tablespoon coconut oil
>
> 1/4 onion, diced
>
> One 15-ounce can organic tomatoes
>
> Fresh basil (optional)

MEATBALLS

> 8 ounces organic ground lamb (Nurturer, substitute organic
>
>   ground turkey and increase to 10 ounces)
>
> 1/4 onion, diced
>
> 1 teaspoon ground cumin
>
> 1 teaspoon ground coriander
>
> 1 teaspoon whole cumin seeds
>
> Pinch of sea salt
>
> 1 tablespoon coconut oil

SALAD

> 1/2 cup cooked quinoa (Nurturer, omit; Ethereal, increase to 1 cup)
>
> 4 Persian cucumbers, chopped
>
> 2 carrots, peeled and sliced into ribbons
>
> 1/4 cup fresh parsley
>
> 2 tablespoons Lemon Vinaigrette (page 210)

Make the tomato sauce: Heat the coconut oil in a medium-sized pan over medium heat. Once the oil coats the pan, add the onion and cook for about two minutes, until browned. Reduce the heat to low and add the tomatoes. Add the fresh basil, if using. Let the tomato sauce simmer while preparing the meatballs.

Make the meatballs: In a medium-sized bowl, combine the lamb, onion, cumin, coriander, cumin seeds, and salt. Mix the ingredients with your hands until the spices are infused into the lamb. Roll the mixture between your hands to make 12 meatballs.

Add the coconut oil to a medium-sized pan over high heat and sear the meatballs for about 4 minutes on each side, until they are cooked to your desired doneness.

Make the salad: Combine the quinoa, cucumbers, carrots, and parsley in a serving bowl. Drizzle with the Lemon Vinaigrette.

Place 6 meatballs on each of two plates. Top with tomato sauce and serve with salad on the side.

CAULIFLOWER RICE BOWL

WONDER WOMAN, FEMME FATALE, AND NURTURER

1 tablespoon olive oil
1 shallot, sliced
2 cups frozen cauliflower rice
$\frac{1}{2}$ cup fresh or frozen corn kernels
Sea salt
2 teaspoons fresh thyme
$\frac{1}{4}$ cup fresh parsley, chopped
3 tablespoons hemp seeds

In a medium pan, heat the olive oil over medium heat. Add the shallot and cook for about 2 minutes, until translucent. Add the cauliflower rice, corn, and a pinch of salt. Sauté for about five minutes, until the vegetables are soft and golden. Add the thyme and parsley. Stir to combine before removing the mixture from the heat. Transfer to a serving bowl and top with hemp seeds. Serve.

DRESSINGS

LEMON VINAIGRETTE

MAKES 4 SERVINGS

Pinch of pink sea salt
2 tablespoons freshly squeezed lemon juice
4 tablespoons extra-virgin olive oil
1 teaspoon Dijon mustard
1 teaspoon raw honey
$1/2$ teaspoon lemon zest
Cracked black pepper

In a mason jar, place the salt, then the lemon juice, followed by 2 tablespoons water and then the olive oil. Add the mustard, honey, lemon zest, and pepper. Shake well until incorporated. Keep refrigerated for up to 2 weeks.

For variety, try adding herbs such as oregano, basil, and chives, diced garlic, or shallots or substitute white balsamic vinegar for the lemon juice.

GREEN GODDESS DRESSING

MAKES 8 SERVINGS

$1/2$ cup avocado

1 small anchovy (optional)

$1/4$ cup coconut milk

1 small garlic clove, chopped

$1/4$ cup chopped fresh parsley

$1/4$ cup chopped fresh tarragon

1 tablespoon chopped fresh chives

$1/2$ tablespoons freshly squeezed lemon juice

2 tablespoons olive oil

Sea salt and freshly cracked black pepper

Put all of the ingredients in the bowl of a blender and blend for 30 seconds until smooth. Add water if the dressing is too thick.

TAHINI DRESSING

Created by Amie Valpone from The Healthy Apple

MAKES 2 SERVINGS

2 tablespoons tahini

Juice of $1/2$ large lemon

1 teaspoon raw honey

1 small garlic clove, minced

Hot water, as needed

Sea salt and freshly cracked black pepper

Whisk together the tahini, lemon juice, honey, garlic, and a few teaspoons hot water in a small bowl. Add more hot water as needed to thin out the dressing to the desired consistency. Season to taste with salt and pepper.

SNACKS

MATCHA GREEN MYLK

WONDER WOMAN, FEMME FATALE, AND ETHEREAL

SERVES 1

12 ounces unsweetened hemp milk
1 teaspoon raw tahini
1/2 teaspoon matcha powder
1 teaspoon coconut sugar
Pinch of pink sea salt
Pinch of ground cinnamon

Place all of the ingredients in a blender and blend until smooth.

PINK MYLK

NURTURER

SERVES 1

12 ounces unsweetened cashew milk
1/2 cup frozen raspberries

1 teaspoon coconut butter

Pinch of pink sea salt

Pinch of vanilla powder or 1 teaspoon vanilla extract

Place all of the ingredients in a blender and blend until smooth.

GOLDEN MYLK

FEMME FATALE

SERVES 1

12 ounces almond or coconut milk

$1/2$ teaspoon ground turmeric powder

$1/4$ teaspoon ground cinnamon

1 teaspoon raw honey

A few grinds of black pepper

Place all of the ingredients in a blender and blend until smooth.

CACAO-INFUSED GOLDEN MYLK

ETHEREAL ONLY

SERVES 1

4 ounces carrot juice

6 ounces almond milk

1 teaspoon ground cinnamon

1 teaspoon cacao powder

1 teaspoon coconut sugar

1 teaspoon coconut oil

Place all of the ingredients in a blender and blend until smooth.

BEET AND CARROT JUICE

ETHEREAL ONLY

SERVES 1

4 ounces carrot juice

4 ounces beet juice

2 ounces filtered water

Squeeze of lemon

Whisk or blend all of the ingredients together until frothy.

GREEN VEGETABLE JUICE

NURTURER AND WONDER WOMAN

SERVES 1

1 large cucumber, peeled and chopped

1/2 small fennel bulb

1/2 pear

2 tablespoons fresh mint leaves (3 or 4 sprigs)

Juice of 1/2 lemon

Put the cucumber, fennel, pear, and mint through a juicer, or place them in the
bowl of a high-speed blender and blend until smooth, adding water to reach

the desired consistency. Add lemon juice to taste, and strain the green vegetable juice if desired.

PINK (OR RUBY RED) GRAPEFRUIT WITH CARAMELIZED COCONUT SUGAR

NURTURER, WONDER WOMAN, AND FEMME FATALE

SERVES 1

1 pink grapefruit (Nurturer, use ruby red grapefruit)
1 teaspoon coconut sugar
1 sprig fresh mint (optional)

Preheat the oven broiler. Cut the grapefruit in half. Place the grapefruit on a baking tray lined with a baking sheet, peel-side down, and sprinkle with the coconut sugar. Place the baking tray with the grapefruit in the oven, keeping the door slightly open so you can watch the fruit. Remove it from the oven when the sugar has caramelized. Sprinkle mint leaves, if using, on top.

NORI WITH CARROT TURMERIC HUMMUS AND AVOCADO

NURTURER, WONDER WOMAN, AND FEMME FATALE

SERVES 1

1 tablespoon Carrot Turmeric Hummus (page 216)
1 nori sheet
¼ avocado, sliced
1 small handful of micro greens

Pinch of sea salt

Pinch of smoked paprika

Spread the hummus in an even layer over the nori sheet, then add the avocado slices and micro greens. Season with salt and paprika.

CARROT TURMERIC HUMMUS

ALL ARCHETYPES

MAKES 12 SERVINGS

3 large carrots

1¹/₂ cups cooked chickpeas

4 tablespoons tahini

1-inch piece of fresh turmeric, peeled

1 teaspoon sea salt

Preheat the oven to 350°F. Rinse, scrub, and cut each carrot into 4 pieces. Place the carrots in an oven-proof dish and roast for 20 minutes. Transfer the carrots to the bowl of a food processor along with the chickpeas, tahini, ¹/₃ cup water, turmeric, and salt and blend until smooth. Add a splash more water or some olive oil if too thick. Store any leftovers in an airtight container in the fridge for up to 1 week.

MISO SOUP

SERVES 1

½ nori sheet, torn into bite-size pieces

2 tablespoons white miso

2 tablespoons hot water

1 cup spinach

1 scallion, sliced

Bring 2 cups water to a boil in a small saucepan over high heat. Add the nori. Reduce the heat and simmer for 5 to 10 minutes. While the seaweed is simmering, combine the miso and the 2 tablespoons hot water in a small bowl. Whisk until the miso is fully broken down. Add the miso and the spinach to the saucepan with the nori. Remove the saucepan from the heat and cover until the spinach wilts. Ladle into a bowl and top with the scallion.

CINNAMON-SPICED PUMPKIN SEEDS

ALL ARCHETYPES

SERVES 8

1 cup pumpkin seeds

1 tablespoon coconut oil

1 tablespoon maple syrup

1 teaspoon ground cinnamon

½ teaspoon ground ginger

¼ teaspoon ground nutmeg

¼ teaspoon smoked paprika

¼ teaspoon sea salt

Preheat the oven to 350°F. In a medium-sized bowl, combine all of the ingredients. Toss to coat the pumpkin seeds, then pour onto a baking pan lined with a baking sheet and spread in an even layer. Roast for 7 minutes or until you can smell the pumpkin seeds toasting. Using a spatula, stir the pumpkin seeds and then roast for 5 minutes more. Remove the pan from the oven and allow the mixture to fully cool before serving. The pumpkin seeds may be stored in an airtight container for up to 1 week.

BLACK SESAME SEED CRACKERS

WONDER WOMAN, FEMME FATALE, AND ETHEREAL

SERVES 4

$\frac{1}{4}$ cup black sesame seeds, ground into a flour in a coffee grinder

$\frac{1}{2}$ cup sunflower seeds

2 tablespoons chia seeds

1 teaspoon sea salt

1 cup gluten-free organic oat flour

$\frac{1}{3}$ cup extra-virgin olive oil

Preheat the oven to 350°F. Place the sesame seed flour, sunflower seeds, chia seeds, salt, and oat flour in a medium-sized bowl and stir until combined. Add $\frac{1}{2}$ cup water and the olive oil and mix to form a dough. Divide the dough into two parts and place them between two sheets of parchment paper. Using a rolling pin (or mason jar), roll out the dough into a thin sheet about $\frac{1}{8}$ inch thick. Remove the top piece of parchment paper and carefully slide the bottom piece of dough with the parchment paper onto a baking pan. Score the dough into desired shapes, cutting about halfway down. Sprinkle with salt. Repeat with the second rolled-out dough.

Bake for 15 to 20 minutes. Remove the baking pan from the oven and flip the whole cracker over onto the baking pan. Don't worry if it breaks. Remove the parchment paper and place the cracker back in the oven for another 10 to 15 minutes or until it's golden on the edges and fully dry. Cool completely. Store in an airtight container for up to 1 week.

CUMIN-SCENTED CHICKPEAS

ETHEREAL ONLY

SERVES 2

One 15-ounce can chickpeas, drained and rinsed
1 tablespoon olive oil
1 teaspoon ground cumin
1 teaspoon fresh thyme
$\frac{1}{2}$ teaspoon smoked paprika
Sea salt to taste

Preheat the oven to 350°F. In a medium bowl, combine the chickpeas, olive oil, cumin, thyme, and paprika and toss to coat. Pour the chickpea mixture onto a baking pan in one layer. Bake for 10 to 15 minutes, until golden brown on the outside but soft on the inside.

SUPERFOOD BARS

ETHEREAL ONLY

Created by my client Jenelle Manzi from the New York City Ballet

SERVES 16

1 cup chopped almonds

³/₄ cup chopped pecans

³/₄ cup pumpkin seeds

¹/₂ cup puffed brown rice, lightly ground

²/₃ cup brown rice syrup

2 tablespoons coconut butter

1 to 2 tablespoons mesquite powder

¹/₄ teaspoon sea salt

1 teaspoon vanilla extract

¹/₃ cup chopped dried mulberries

3 tablespoons cacao nibs

Preheat the oven to 350°F. Line a 9 x 9-inch glass baking dish with parchment paper.

Mix the almonds, pecans, pumpkin seeds, and puffed rice together in a large bowl. Using a double boiler or saucepan over medium heat, warm and blend the rice syrup, coconut butter, mesquite powder, salt, and vanilla until smooth and caramel-like. Spoon the mixture over the dry ingredients. Add the mulberries and cacao nibs and mix with your hands until fully combined.

Press the mixture into the prepared baking dish. Bake for 10 to 12 minutes. Let cool slightly and cut into 16 rectangular bars.

SUNFLOWER-SEED CRACKERS WITH TAHINI

ETHEREAL ONLY

SERVES 4

½ cup sunflower seeds, ground into a flour

½ cup chia seeds

½ cup pumpkin seeds

1 tablespoon fresh thyme

1½ teaspoons fresh rosemary

Sea salt

1 tablespoon tahini, for serving

Put the flour, chia seeds, pumpkin seeds, thyme, and rosemary in a medium-sized bowl. Add ¾ to 1 cup water slowly, combining the mixture until it forms a dough. Let sit for 5 minutes. If it gets too dry, add more water, but it should not be sitting in water.

Preheat the oven to 350°F. Divide the dough into two parts and place between two sheets of parchment paper. Using a rolling pin (or mason jar), roll out the dough into a thin sheet about ⅛ inch thick. Remove the top piece of parchment and carefully slide the bottom piece of the dough with the parchment onto a baking pan. Score the dough into desired shapes, cutting about halfway down. Sprinkle with salt. Repeat with the second rolled-out dough.

Bake for 15 to 20 minutes. Remove the baking pan from the oven and flip the whole cracker over onto the baking pan. Don't worry if it breaks. Remove the parchment paper and place the cracker back in the oven for another 10 to 15 minutes or until it's golden on the edges and fully dry. Cool completely.

Break the crackers into shapes and serve a handful with 1 tablespoon of tahini. Store the leftover crackers in an airtight container for up to 2 weeks at room temperature.

CACAO, COCONUT, AND GOJI BERRY TRAIL MIX

ETHEREAL ONLY

SERVES 1

1 tablespoon goji berries
1 tablespoon unsweetened flaked coconut
1 tablespoon cacao nibs
1 tablespoon chopped macadamia nuts

Mix the goji berries, coconut, cacao nibs, and macadamia nuts in a small bowl and enjoy.

CHOCOLATE COCONUT CHIA SEED PUDDING

ETHEREAL ONLY

SERVES 1

3 tablespoons chia seeds
4 ounces almond milk
4 ounces coconut milk
1 tablespoon cacao
1 teaspoon maple syrup
Splash of vanilla extract

1 tablespoon cacao nibs
Unsweetened coconut flakes

Place the chia seeds, almond milk, coconut milk, cacao, maple syrup, and vanilla in a mason jar and shake vigorously until the seeds are fully submerged in the liquid. Let the mixture sit for 15 minutes. Shake once more and top with the cacao nibs and coconut before serving.

CITRUS-MINT SALAD

WONDER WOMAN

SERVES 1

$^1/_2$ pink grapefruit
1 blood orange or tangerine
1 teaspoon coconut sugar
2 tablespoons sliced fresh mint leaves

Peel the grapefruit and orange and cut them horizontally, perpendicular to the segments, to create wheels. Place them in a small serving bowl and toss with the coconut sugar and mint leaves.

BERRY-MINT SALAD

NURTURER

SERVES 1

$^1/_2$ cup blueberries
$^1/_2$ cup raspberries

Squeeze of lime juice

4 fresh mint leaves, torn

10 pistachios, chopped

Place the blueberries and raspberries in a small bowl. Add the lime juice and mint and toss together. Sprinkle with the pistachios and serve.

COCONUT MACAROONS

ALL ARCHETYPES

SERVES 6

$\frac{1}{2}$ cup unsweetened coconut flakes

$\frac{1}{4}$ cup almond flour

1 tablespoon coconut oil

1 tablespoon maple syrup

1 teaspoon vanilla extract

Pinch of sea salt

Place all of the ingredients in the bowl of a food processor and pulse until well combined. Use a tablespoon to roll the mixture into 6 balls. Refrigerate for 30 minutes before eating. Store leftovers in an airtight container in the refrigerator for up to 1 week.

CACAO MATCHA TRUFFLES

ETHEREAL ONLY

SERVES 8

¹/₂ cup hemp seeds

¹/₂ cup hazelnuts

2 tablespoons cacao powder

¹/₄ teaspoon ground cinnamon

Pinch of ground cardamom

12 dates, pitted*

2 tablespoons coconut oil

1 teaspoon matcha powder, such as Cap Beauty Matcha

Place the hemp seeds, hazelnuts, cacao powder, cinnamon, and cardamom in the bowl of a food processor and pulse until the nuts and seeds are broken into a rough flour. Add the dates and coconut oil. Continue to pulse until the mixture forms a thick dough. If too thick to combine, add water 1 tablespoon at a time until you reach the desired consistency. Remove the mixture from the food processor and use a tablespoon to roll the dough into 8 balls. Refrigerate for 30 minutes before dusting with matcha powder and serving.

*If the dates are not soft, place them in a bowl and cover with boiling water. Let sit for 5 minutes before using. Save the soaking liquid if needed later in the recipe.

CHOCOLATE ALMOND MILK

FEMME FATALE

SERVES 1

12 ounces unsweetened almond milk

2 teaspoons cacao

1 teaspoon coconut oil

1 teaspoon maple syrup

$1/4$ teaspoon ground cinnamon

Place all of the ingredients in the bowl of a blender and blend until smooth. If desired, warm in a small saucepan over low heat.

FIG AND COCONUT BALLS

WONDER WOMAN, FEMME FATALE, AND ETHEREAL

SERVES 8

$1/2$ cup dried figs, de-stemmed (Femme Fatale, substitute dried apricots)

$1/2$ cup unsweetened coconut flakes

$1/4$ cup cashew pieces

$1/4$ teaspoon ground cinnamon

Pinch of sea salt

Soften the figs by placing them in a medium-sized bowl and pouring simmering water over them. Let sit for 5 minutes while preparing the rest of the recipe.

Place the coconut, cashew pieces, cinnamon, and salt in the bowl of a food processor and pulse until a flour starts to form. Drain the figs and add to the processor. Continue to pulse until the mixture forms a thick dough. Remove the mixture from the food processor and use a tablespoon to roll the mixture into 9 balls. Refrigerate for 30 minutes before serving.

THE SIX Rs
TO HEAL
YOUR MIND

You'll recall that the foundation of the Archetype Model is breaking the cycle that determines your eating behaviors:

SOURCE OF SELF-WORTH ➡ CHANGE IN BEHAVIORS ➡
CHANGE IN EATING BEHAVIORS

While Part II addressed the dietary part, in order for this new way of eating and thinking about food to stick, it's essential that you examine the genesis of this cycle—*why* you want to eat as you do in the first place. Without addressing the why, you'll constantly berate yourself for not being able to follow a prescribed eating plan. You'll jump from one diet to the next, hoping that some magical formula will save you. Your salvation is found in your mind. If you want peace with food, you need to understand all of the factors that influence your behaviors—not just *what* you do but *why* you make certain choices and behave the way you do.

The Archetype Model draws on several foundational psychological models to explain the reasons behind your actions. In psychology, there are four primary schools of thought when it comes to how we make decisions. First, there is the Darwinian model, which holds that we are genetically and evolutionarily programmed to behave in a certain way. When it comes to food, we see our genes at work in our basic body shape—are we a curvy Nurturer or a naturally thin Ethereal?—and how we process food—are you genetically programmed to eat sweets after a stress response?[1] Are you more sensitive to bitter foods and therefore crave sweetness?[2] Don't worry, you don't need to know if you have these genes in order to alter your taste preferences. What you eat is more important than your genes, since food (along with your environment) acts as the trigger that switches off and on the expression of your genes. This is known as epigenetics—how your environment reacts with your genes—and is what prevents poor genetics from becoming your destiny. I simply want you to understand that your genes and biochemistry (which we covered in prior chapters) can influence your food choices.

The second behavioral model comes from Abraham Maslow. You might be familiar with Maslow from his famous Hierarchy of Needs theory, which posits that human beings must fulfill basic needs like food, health, and safety before they can turn their attention toward "higher" needs like love and self-esteem. Maslow believed that humans are not simply preprogrammed machines who behave solely out of genetics or instinct but rather autonomous beings endowed with free will who are constantly trying to reach their full potential, which Maslow called self-actualization. According to Maslow, our ability to make decisions is governed by what we call willpower. If you have the desire to achieve something, you'll start making behavioral changes that lead you toward your goal—like starting the archetype meal plan to achieve weight loss. But, as you know, willpower isn't always enough to sustain you. Further, I believe there's a bidirectional relationship at work within Maslow's Hierarchy of Needs; your food choices depend on your self-esteem just as your self-esteem depends on your food choices. If your self-esteem is poor, your food choices are likely to be poor as well. If you're struggling to stay on a diet, it does not mean you have no willpower. It simply means there are other equally strong forces at work.

One of those forces is the Pavlovian response, that is, your habits. Psychologist Ivan Pavlov revolutionized our understanding of behavior with his famous experiment in which he got a dog to associate the ringing of a bell with the arrival of food. By doing so, Pavlov conditioned the dog to engage in a behavior (in this case, salivating) that was not directed by evolution, thus proving that the brain could be rewired to unconsciously associate a neutral stimulus—like the ringing of a bell—with a previously unrelated reward—like a delicious meal. If you automatically reach for a glass of wine the second you come home from work or start to crave chocolate at three p.m., you already know how this stimulus-response pattern has affected your eating behaviors.

Darwin, Maslow, and Pavlov all provide different but equally valid insights into how we make decisions—not only about what to eat but about everything else in our lives: the types of relationships we form, the type of work we do, our daily patterns, and our responses to novel experiences. But it was another psychologist, Carl Jung, who identified the fourth factor that directs our behavior—our unconscious.

Certain experiences, usually those from childhood, reside in our unconscious mind and influence how we perceive the world. Jung, the founder of Analytical psychology, believed that the unconscious mind was a more potent driver of our behaviors than the conscious mind. He proposed that bringing conscious awareness to the unconscious was essential for wholeness. Archetypes are used for insight into the unconscious.

As you are familiar, women who share the same archetype source their self-worth from the same place; however, the situations that each woman experiences will be different. The purpose of this section is to help you bring to consciousness the memories that are lodged into your unconscious and are influencing your behavior. You cannot change these experiences, but you can change your interpretation of them, your judgment of them, and the shame you may have unwittingly attached to them. From here you'll be better prepared to move through the rest of the behavior cycle and will find it easier to alter the patterns that have caused you to fall out of balance.

FACTORS THAT INFLUENCE OUR CHOICES

PROMINENT FIGURE	CAUSE	EFFECT
DARWIN	Genetics/Epigenetics	You eat a muffin because of low blood-sugar levels.
MASLOW	Free Will/Willpower	You start a diet or detox because you want to lose weight.
PAVLOV	Habits	You eat M&M's at three p.m. every day.
JUNG	Unconscious	You crave ice cream because you equate it with love and bonding from your childhood summer vacations

THE SIX Rs

My clients are smart, educated, and highly motivated women, and many are already familiar with some of the basic psychology surrounding human behavior. But unless these women have taken the time to reflect on their behaviors, they are not likely to be aware of how the four psychological drivers of decision making—the evolutionary, motivational, habitual, and unconscious—are influencing their inability to condition themselves to eat cauliflower instead of candy. Getting there is a six-step process that I refer to as the Six Rs. Each R represents a different piece of the decision-making puzzle:

1. Restore
2. Recognize
3. Reinterpret
4. Release
5. Rewire
6. Revive

The following chapters will examine each of the Six Rs and provide tools and exercises to help you work through them in turn. Restore refers to the epigenetic aspect that restores the mind to peak condition.

The next three Rs—Recognize, Reinterpret, and Release—all relate to the unconscious mind. Working through each of these will help you identify the core childhood memories that are directing your behavior so that you can rewrite the script that has been limiting your life. You can't fight a monster that you can't see, so this step is critical to achieving lasting change.

This process is the most complex aspect of the Six Rs, and it is also the most essential. Don't expect to complete this stage in a couple of hours and consider yourself "cured." This is an ongoing process; you did not become who you are overnight, nor will you change who you are overnight. Be patient and compassionate with yourself and know that at the end of this journey lies the freedom from the misguided beliefs that have caused you to struggle for so long.

Once you see how your unconscious mind is affecting your behaviors, you can take practical steps to change those behaviors for good. This involves Rewiring your brain to develop new habits and rid yourself of old ones. Our brains are incredibly powerful. Up until now, you have been using that power to shore up unconscious but mistaken beliefs and protect yourself from repeating the negative emotions associated with those childhood memories. Once you've identified and reinterpreted these beliefs, you can redirect your brainpower to your benefit.

The final stage in the process comes when you Revive yourself by harnessing all of your feminine energies. This is where your archetype takes a backseat in order to make room for the positive qualities of the other archetypes, enabling you to ascend to your crown. In psychological terms you are, as Abraham Maslow suggested, "self-actualizing," and reaching your full potential. Not only will you be in balance physically and emotionally, but you will have become the woman you most want to be and an inspiration for others.

As one of my clients, Kelly, a recovering out-of-balance Wonder Woman, said, "I just can't believe how much energy I was wasting on feeling guilty, thinking I was impoverished, being pissed at everything . . . the list just goes on. I've realized how powerful my thoughts are—the good as well as the ugly. I now find myself listening to music, going on longer runs, watching and listening to my daughter play pretend with her dolls, and enjoying warm hugs and kisses from my husband. I can finally take in all the glory of being a mother, wife, and friend. But it has even more far-reaching repercussions. My daughter is picking up on my vibe, too, and she's becoming a more loving and conscious role model. I started this journey for myself but realize it is much larger than me. It's breaking the feeling of entrapment and unworthiness passed down through my family's mother/daughter relationships for generations."

CHAPTER 15

Restore Your Brain

———

Next to diet, stress is one of the main reasons we put on—or struggle to lose—weight. If you read the chapter on Wonder Woman, you saw how this connection shows up physically when the body produces too much cortisol and directs the storage of fat to the belly. But stress also heightens our emotional response, which can impede our ability to make good decisions, including how we eat and respond to events. That's why the first of the Six Rs is to restore your mind so it is better prepared to process stressful situations, emotions, and thoughts. This is critical, not only so you can handle everyday stresses but also so you can manage the challenging process of examining your childhood experiences and reclaiming your self-worth.

We have already covered one critical way to restore your mind through the meal plans and food recommendations I provided in Parts I and II. By following these guidelines, you will give your brain the nutrients it needs to thrive and will be rewarded with improved focus, mood, and energy. But food is only one solution. Sleep, meditation, movement, and sound currents are also powerful catalysts toward bringing the mind back into balance.

To understand how these tools work, it's important to understand the role that stress plays in your life. The stress hormones—cortisol, adrenaline, and noradrenaline—are often perceived as harmful. I'm frequently asked, "Aren't they why I feel stressed?" Not exactly. It's your *perception* of the stressors that makes you feel stressed. The stress hormones activate physical changes in the body to keep you from crumbling into an emotional mess. For instance, if you're bitten by a dog, stress hormones will send blood to your arms and legs so you can quickly escape and make it to the emergency room. They also activate mental acuity so you can explain to the nurse what happened and get treatment quickly. Without these stress hormones, your response would be lackluster, and any small perturbation, like someone accidentally knocking into you on the street, would cause inconsolable weeping.

The catch is, you need just the right amount of stress hormones. Too much and you'll feel anxious and start to gain weight on your belly, as Wonder Women often do; too little and you'll feel overwhelmed, exhausted, and despondent, unable to navigate life's up and downs with any sense of ease and vitality. Because stress hormones help turn body fat into energy, having too few leads to slow weight loss; you'll feel like nothing is budging even though you're doing everything right!

There are five different types of stress. Some of these are triggered by external factors over which we have little or no control. In these moments, our stress response is extremely helpful because it allows us to respond to these events with urgency. Others, however, come from within and, with the right mental tools at our disposal, we can learn to limit their effects.

1. Sudden emergencies such as rushing your child to the emergency room, your house being burglarized, or a truck swerving into your lane;
2. Major life stressors such as a death in the family, a health or financial crisis, or a divorce;

3. Trivial irritations like a traffic jam, your partner not making the bed, or an incompetent customer service rep;

4. False interpretations such as perception of self, feeling trapped, being overwhelmed; and lastly,

5. Unresolved psychological traumas from your childhood or secrets from your past.

While you want your adrenal glands to respond quickly in an emergency, you don't need them firing off copious amounts of stress hormones when you are dealing with trivial irritations, false interpretations, and unresolved traumas. The more negative your view of these internal stressors, the more rapidly you'll deplete your reserves of cortisol, adrenaline, and noradrenaline, leaving you even less prepared to handle actual stressors like emergencies or major life events should they arise.

The stealthiest stressors are unresolved psychological traumas. According to the Adverse Childhood Experiences (ACE) study, which discovered connections between childhood traumas and health and interpersonal problems in adulthood, it's the day-to-day minor traumas you experience as a child—not a one-off traumatic event—that predict chronic disease later in life.[1] It's feeling ignored by a parent, excluded from the girl gang, not feeling pretty enough, or being humiliated in front of the class.

When something threatens your sense of self-worth even years afterward, you will become triggered, whether you realize it or not, because the event subconsciously reminds you of adverse experiences from your childhood. The stress we feel in these situations elicits an emotional response that can alter your behavior, often in unproductive ways. Your stress hormones will be supercharged. We see this in the Nurturer who comfort-eats when she senses she has disappointed someone. Or the Wonder Woman who crumbles after receiving criticism on her work and needs a Xanax (or glass of wine) to calm down. Or the Femme Fatale who feels like the fattest person in the room at a gallery opening—and then goes home and binge-eats. Or the Ethereal who is dismissed for being "spacey" and then retreats into isolation, becoming even more disconnected from those around her.

By restoring your physical brain to its optimal health, through diet and the practices below, you give it the energy and clarity it needs to help you on your journey toward becoming a more peaceful and resilient version of you.

SLEEP

Quality sleep is critical to restoring both the body and the mind. Researchers have found that insufficient sleep increases hunger, food intake, and inflammation—all factors that can contribute to weight gain. In one study, women who got between four and seven hours of sleep for four consecutive nights ate 400 more calories per day than they did on days where they got eight hours of sleep.[2] This is partially due to how the brain responds to foods when we are tired. Researchers have noticed more activity in the reward and hedonic areas of the brain and less activity in that rational processing part of the brain when sleep was shortened.[3] Insufficient sleep can set you up for overeating . . . and it won't be for broccoli! To make matters worse, lack of sleep destabilizes the way you regulate your glucose levels; if you grab a gluten-free muffin on the way to work because you overslept, that carb-loaded breakfast will cause your body to release even more insulin—thus blocking the fat-burning process—than it would if you had gotten more rest.

In another study, lack of sleep caused the hunger hormone, ghrelin, to increase by 28 percent and the appetite-suppressing hormone, leptin, to drop by 18 percent.[4] Not enough sleep makes you hungrier because two appetite-regulating hormones go out of balance. Adding to that, shortened sleep increases inflammatory mediators such as tumor necrosis factor alpha (TNFα), interleukin-1 (IL-1), and interleukin-6 (IL-6).[5] This kind of chronic inflammation makes it even harder to lose weight.

Cortisol is even higher the evening following partial sleep deprivation.[6] A Wonder Woman is the most prone to skipping sleep, unconsciously fearing that if she doesn't respond to those emails immediately, she'll feel the wrath of a boss who expected more from her. What's worse, she's read countless articles in which extremely successful people boast of sleeping six hours or less a night and she assumes she must do the same if she wants to achieve on their level. Just to be clear: financial or professional success doesn't necessarily mean healthy. The brain functions exponentially faster after a good night's sleep.

It's not just the amount of sleep you get; the type and depth of sleep also matters. Your mental agility and cognitive processing are much quicker if you get a deeper level of sleep, allowing you to make smarter and clearer decisions.

What's more, you make mental connections and process emotional experiences from the day during REM (rapid eye movement) sleep, also known as dream sleep. When REM sleep is disrupted, these memories can remain unprocessed and filter in and out of your subconscious during your waking hours, subtly influencing your behavior. You'll know when your REM sleep was disrupted because you'll be irritable, excessively focused on the negative, and distrustful of others the next day. This occurs because the anterior cingulate (which mediates empathy, intuition, and social awareness) is most active during the REM sleep cycle, and if REM is reduced, so, too, is the ability to regulate your emotions and maintain a positive outlook on life. If you take a sleeping aid that inhibits the REM cycle, it's going to be harder for you to process experiences from the day objectively and investigate the behavioral patterns that make you feel stuck and despondent (and are probably part of the cause of the insomnia). Fortunately, there are some very easy and simple tricks to help you capture more sleep, and specifically REM sleep.

When a good night's sleep is simply not possible—your kids were up all night, you were anxious, you finished that report at three a.m.—don't get stressed about it (that just makes it worse!). Be aware that your brain is functioning below capacity and stay vigilant about cutting carbs and skipping sweets, since your body can't regulate its glucose levels well on such diminished sleep reserves. Yes, it will be difficult since you'll be up against appetite and brain changes, but your mind is more powerful than any biochemical process. If the voice in your head says, "I'm so tired; I *need* that muffin," simply acknowledge that you're tired and what you *really* need is sleep. Get to bed earlier that night and you'll wake up the next day with a brighter outlook, grateful that you didn't overindulge in carbs because you were tired.

SLEEP SOLUTIONS FOR EVERY ARCHETYPE

Getting a good night's sleep—at least 7.5 hours—is essential for weight loss and fighting fatigue, but what if you can't sleep or wake up frequently throughout the night? Certain nutrients and breath practices can help. Start with these six tips:

1. Before bed, take 300 mg of magnesium glycinate to help calm the mind.
2. Before bed, take 50 mg of 5-HTP, which is the precursor to serotonin and melatonin. If you are taking an SSRI, this should only be taken under your physician's guidance.
3. Wear a silk eye mask to block out any light, as light switches off melatonin.
4. Engage in a five-minute calming breath series. Lie on your bed on your on stomach with the right side of your face on

the pillow. Set your alarm for five minutes. Close your eyes. Hold your right nostril so you breathe through your left nostril. Breathing through the left nostril is calming, while breathing through the right is stimulating. Breathe in and out through the left nostril for five minutes and allow your mind to relax and drift off.

5. Use a sleep meditation app such as aSleep, Simply Being, and Sleepmaker Rain.

6. Check your vitamin D levels. Low vitamin D has been associated with shortened REM sleep. Take 2,000 IU of vitamin D daily until your levels are restored.

MEDITATION

Meditation is just as important as the food you put into your mouth. It enables you to become more intuitive, more compassionate, and to fear less, ruminate less, and be more emotionally resilient. Meditation has the ability to change the physiology of the brain, allowing you to release past traumas and dysfunctional emotions. Consistent meditation stimulates the growth of new neurons and increases blood flow to the anterior cingulate, which acts as a conduit between the prefrontal cortex (your rational mind) and the amygdala (the emotional center of the brain). When you're angry or upset, the activity in the prefrontal cortex becomes reduced, so you might not realize that you are acting irrationally. The activity in the amygdala becomes exaggerated, making it nearly impossible for you to listen to another person, let alone feel compassion or empathy. Meditation changes the direction of this activity—away from the amygdala toward the prefrontal cortex—so your mind becomes more expansive and illuminated and you can stop responding from a primitive program of fear.

Chronically elevated cortisol levels physically shrink the prefrontal cortex and the hippocampus (where memory is stored and accessed). Yet a twenty-minute meditation has repeatedly been shown to lower cortisol, even in new meditators, thereby restoring the brain's functionality.[7] Meditation also activates six hundred genes that regulate the stress response and this is, no doubt, why consistent meditators recover more quickly from stressful situations and can easily "switch off" stress.[8] In another study, daily meditation for eight weeks changed the brain regions associated with memory, empathy, sense of self, and stress.[9] Meditation is a powerful catalyst in changing the physiology of your brain, thereby directing you to live physically healthier and with joy and love.

Not surprisingly, food and meditation work in concert. A clean diet makes you want to meditate. A poor diet makes you resistant to meditation. Meditation also helps to reduce addictive patterns (food, relationships, and negative thoughts). When one of my binge-eating clients meditated in the morning, she could say no to her nighttime online ordering, but when she skipped a day, she'd find herself hijacked by the call of ice cream and cookies at midnight. Research also supports this. When a group of obese women meditated for twenty minutes every day for six weeks, their binge eating decreased by a whopping 60 percent![10]

Meditation isn't a "nice to-do," nor is it something you do when you can "fit it in." You need to prioritize meditating as you do brushing your teeth. I recommend making meditation the first thing you do upon waking and before you check social media and emails. This is when your mind is most receptive since the brain waves are still at a lower frequency following hours of sleep. Start with a ten-minute meditation and increase to twenty minutes when your schedule allows.

The benefits of meditation are cumulative. While you'll feel serene as you emerge from your meditation, the more consistent your practice, the more you'll find your day-to-day emotional responses becoming less reactive because you've changed where the brain responds from under stress. You'll respond in a calm, centered, and graceful way. You'll have clarity on the situation. You'll see the truth.

How to Meditate

Meditation is not a religion. It is a practice designed to settle and restore your mind. Unless you're practicing Zen meditation, the goal of meditation isn't to have zero thoughts; it's to decrease the excitation of the brain waves. Emily Fletcher, meditation teacher and founder of *The M-word*, explains that you can't stop your thoughts just as you can't stop your heart from beating. What you can control, though, is the frequency of the brain waves, moving them from a high, active learning state to a receptive low-wave theta state. All you need to do is stop judging yourself for having thoughts during your meditation practice or telling yourself you "can't" meditate. Just as you can breathe in and out, your mind can focus and expand. Expansion will happen naturally as long you don't attempt to control it.

When I first started meditating, my mind was very reluctant to submit to the "nothingness" of meditation. I would squirm in my seat, wondering how I could possibly make it through the next twenty minutes. Subconsciously, part of me feared that meditation might make me more passive and blunt my innate sharpness (Wonder Woman!). I soon discovered that meditation actually opened me up to a dynamic "nothingness," a profound stillness that revealed truth and clarity within myself and others. My mind became razor sharp at slicing through false beliefs, and I found myself stripping away delusional thoughts like peeling back the layers of an onion. I now relish those twenty minutes of tranquility and consider it my time to reconnect to the magnificence of life.

If you're scared to try meditation because you don't think you'll be good at it or you've tried it but given up because your mind wouldn't settle, you may need a little help. I highly recommend you use sound currents, such as music, mantras, or the harmonics of a gong, to help facilitate the relaxation response. Guided meditations and mantra-based meditations all use intentional sound currents that can help change the frequency of your brain waves. Just as there are different types of exercise, there are different types of meditation, and I encourage you to try out different forms to see which one is the most effective for you. Biet Simkin, a dear friend and esteemed meditation teacher, has kindly created a ten-minute guided meditation for you. This can be found at my website, danajames.com.

MOVEMENT

Movement has been shown to increase a chemical called brain-derived neurotrophic factor (BDNF), which tells the brain to produce new brain cells. Only when new brain cells are created can you break habits. Exercise is not just for reshaping the body, it's for reshaping the brain. The exercise recommendations provided in your archetype's chapter will not only help you burn fat and tone your muscles; they'll also help you sharpen your mind.

Tony Robbins, the renowned self-help and motivational speaker, says, "Motion changes emotion." In other words, move the body when you don't feel good. Jump up and down for three minutes like a two-year-old throwing a temper tantrum when your mind is in a tug-of-war telling you to eat (and not eat) that cookie. I promise you, the movement will make your desire dwindle and you will find it much easier to say no. Part of the reason that movement works is that it disperses the body's stress hormones. If you have ever seen a dog that has just been in a fight, you may have noticed it shook its body vigorously afterward. The dog instinctively knows how to release its stress hormones. Humans need to do the same.

Taryn Toomey, creator of *The Class by Taryn Toomey*, has created a sixty-minute movement class that all the archetypes will find beneficial. It combines movement with an emotional release and is specifically designed to shed the emotional layers that hold you back from living your fullest life. You can do just ten minutes as a tool for emotional release or the entire class for a physical and mind-altering experience. You'll find at instructions at danajames.com.

SOUND CURRENTS

Sound currents include music, mantras, chanting, singing, the beat of a drum, and even your own voice. Different beats, melodies, and tones can instantly change your emotional state. Think about how you feel when you listen to classical music versus R&B. They create a different mood. Similarly, the music you play to get ready for a night out isn't likely to be the same music you play when you want Sunday chill-out vibes. One reason movement and meditation are so effective in changing your emotions is their use of sound. If you are not in a place where exercise or meditation is feasible, you can use sound to quickly change how you feel. You can put on music, chant, sing, or scream it out (just not at others). I can't think of a client ever reporting that she binged while listening to music she enjoyed or after meditating and chanting for ten minutes.

I frequently recommend that my clients listen to calming music on the way home from work as a way to transition out of work mode and into mother or lover mode. If they bring the intensity of the hectic workday into the home, they can find themselves eating with the same frenzy they use to tackle their day. Calming music helps facilitate this transformation, which requires a different set of personality traits—patience and playfulness, not tenacity and temerity.

Using these four tools—sleep, meditation, movement, and sound currents—together with your archetype meal plan, you will prime your brain to create new neural connections so new habits can easily be formed. The next step is to go deeper into the psychology behind your repetitive behaviors. These behaviors may be as mindless as constant overeating, but if this is out of alignment with who you want to be, it can distract you from living an enriched and fulfilled life. No woman should be robbed of that, particularly when it's her mind that's the thief.

CHAPTER 16

Recognize Your Core Memories

The second R—Recognize—is loosely inspired by cognitive behavioral therapy (CBT), a psychotherapy model that seeks to identify the root cause of behaviors rather than simply attempting to alter those behaviors. The CBT model asserts that your *thoughts* drive your emotions, your body's physical response, and your behavior. For example, if you had plans to have dinner with a friend and she canceled at the last minute, how would you feel? Here are three possible reactions:

1. You might think, "She does this to me all the time. She's such a flake. Why am I still friends with her?" This train of thought may cause three things to happen:

   a. Emotion—You feel angry.
   b. Physical—Your adrenaline spikes.
   c. Behavior—You shove cookies in your mouth to cope with the anger.

2. You might think, "Oh no, did I do something wrong? Does she not like me? Did I do something to upset her?" With these thoughts, three things might happen:

    a. Emotion—You feel sad.

    b. Physical—Your serotonin levels drop.

    c. Behavior—You shove cookies in your mouth to cope with the sadness.

3. You might think, "Oh, I hope she's okay, but I'm actually glad I don't have to go out. I was feeling like I needed a night to myself. Now I can stay in, take a bath, and finish that novel." With this thought, three things might happen:

    a. Emotion—You feel elated.

    b. Physical—Your dopamine levels spike.

    c. Behavior—You do something kind for yourself.

As you can see, it's not the situation that has caused the emotional, physical, and behavioral responses but the *interpretation* of the event. If you want to change your behavior, you'll need to reinterpret the events that lead to those feelings and behaviors, which is exactly what we do in the third R—Reinterpret. But before you can do that, you must delve into your mind to recognize the memories that are shaping your behavior today.

The most influential memories are those that were formed before you turned eighteen, when your prefrontal cortex (which processes logic and reasoning) had not yet reached its full development. That means you viewed your childhood and teenage experiences through the lens of how they made you feel, not through rational thought. And because emotions enhance the encoding of a memory in the brain, you'll remember these memories more vividly than those that have been interpreted logically. Unless you recognize these memories, you won't be able to reinterpret them through the more rational perspective you've developed as an adult.

To illustrate just how profound an effect your childhood memories have on your behavior today, I want to introduce you to my client Emily. Emily and I had been working together for several months, and she'd lost the first twenty pounds quickly by following the program outlined in this book. But the last ten pounds were proving more challenging. She was stuck in a familiar pattern of weekday weight loss and weekend weight gain. The behavior part was pretty obvious: she'd diet during the week, only to blow it on the weekend. On Friday night she'd drive to her home in upstate New York, where her friends had pizza and wine waiting for her. Emily obviously knew that routinely indulging in pizza and wine wasn't going to help her lose weight, but she felt compelled to join in and eat and drink whatever was on offer. Starting her weekend off on that note quickly spiraled into "all-or-nothing" thinking; having already "blown" her diet, she'd eat and drink her way through the weekend with gusto, gaining back several pounds in the process.

While I'm all for a celebration with friends, Emily's behavior wasn't celebratory. It was compulsive and addictive. Once the food and alcohol were in front of her, she couldn't resist them. During the week, however, she was completely in control. I nonchalantly said to Emily, "Why don't you just let your friends know that you don't want pizza and you'll pick up dinner before you leave the city?" I reasoned that if she could change her Friday night meal, her weekend eating might improve. When I looked at her I saw tears in her eyes. With a quavering voice she confessed, "Dana, I just don't know if I can do that." Emily is a stoic Wonder Woman who rarely expresses emotion, so I knew we'd stumbled onto something big: something that was going to lead to Emily's breakthrough. Tears mean truth.

I asked Emily what image had just flashed before her to cause the tears. Emily said she saw herself as a distressed eight-year-old who'd gone to school one day and discovered she had been ostracized by the other girls in her class. She felt rejected, sad, and humiliated, and this isolation went on for an entire year. Not wanting *ever* to feel this way again, Emily's mind naturally prompted her to avoid any situation that might cause her to be excluded, including the simple act of saying no to food when she was with friends. Emily's need to be part of the "gang," whether it was the girl gang, the work gang, or the Friday-night-pizza gang, trumped her desire to stick to her diet.

Emily wasn't consciously thinking of her childhood exclusion memory when she was eating pizza with her friends, and that's the issue. The mind doesn't show you the memory behind your self-sabotaging behaviors. Only when I inquired about her tears was Emily able to connect the two. Her self-sabotaging food behavior was all an effort to protect herself from potential rejection.

Not being able to say no to pizza with her friends was not the only protective behavior Emily had adopted as a response to this memory. It spilled over into her career and marriage. At work, she embraced the Wonder Woman habit of perfection, attempting to circumvent criticism in an effort to protect herself from being fired. While losing one's job is never pleasant, it would have been especially traumatic for Emily because she would have relived the pain she felt as a rejected eight-year-old child. In her marriage, she exhausted herself to become the "perfect" wife, believing that if she was the perfect wife, her husband could not possibly leave her. Emily, like most other Wonder Women, also wanted to look good, and carrying extra weight meant she was less than perfect. Lucky for Emily, her desire to lose weight gave her the opportunity to heal these emotional scars and transform her life into something richer and bolder, free from fear of rejection. While losing weight doesn't create a new life, the process of unpacking the memories that inhibit the weight loss does.

Emily's childhood memory is what I call a "core memory" because it was at the *core* of her subconscious behaviors. These core memories will lay down the foundation for your archetype and very often for your eating behavior as well, just as they had in Emily's case. After the incident in elementary school, Emily needed to find a way to fit in. She engaged in the protective patterns of perfection and passivity (the amplification and withdrawal of her Wonder Woman archetype) so as not to open herself up to further rejection. She also made sure she did everything to ensure her inclusion in any group, which in the case of her weekend friends included dysfunctional eating behaviors.

RECOGNIZING YOUR CORE MEMORIES

Your core memories are usually tucked into the darkest depths of the unconscious, but until they are unearthed, you can't change the meaning you've attached to them. You'll find yourself repeating the same defective patterns over and over again. Sigmund Freud called this "repetition compulsion," which is the attempt by the unconscious to repeat what is unresolved until we get it right. By bringing these core memories to your conscious mind—by recognizing them—you can reinterpret them so you can adjust your behaviors, your body's physical response, and your emotional response. As Joe Dispenza, neuroscientist and author of *Breaking the Habit of Being Yourself*, says, "Memories without an emotional charge are wisdom."

Core memories are accessed through a series of questions. These memories usually have some shame attached to them, which is why you hide them in the depths of your psyche. They may be relatively minor and you might wonder, "How can *these* be influencing me today?" Let me tell you, they are.

When you review the questions in the exercise on page 253, your mind is likely to respond in pictures. Don't analyze or judge your answers. Just write down as many memories as you can think of. Don't judge the memories; they are all relevant. The logical mind may brush off a memory as insignificant, but if it came to you, it's not. You have remembered it for a reason. All you are doing is taking thoughts from your subconscious and unconscious mind to your conscious mind. You're bringing them out of hiding.

Once you've collected these memories, there will be one or two that feel highly emotional. These are your core memories, the mother memories of which future memories will bear the imprint. For instance, if you have a specific memory of feeling neglected, you will interpret later experiences through this feeling and carry those interpretations with you as you move through life. You might feel neglected in your intimate relationships and in friendships, and feel unheard at work. These later memories reinforce the feelings triggered by the core memory. However, once you crack the core memory, it's like changing your DNA—the later memories carry much less of an emotional sting.

Start with questions related to your archetype, and if you want extra credit (Wonder Woman, you probably will), see if any of the other archetypes' questions resonate with you. Because of society's focus on female looks, I suspect many of you will have experiences that apply to the Femme Fatale. Write those memories down, too.

One important proviso: If you have suffered a severe trauma in your life like abuse, abandonment, addiction, or mental illness, you should consult with a licensed therapist to help you work through these experiences. Trauma alters our brain so profoundly that it can be difficult to work through the mental exercises on your own. Don't be afraid to ask for help.

EXERCISE

THE MEMORIES

Use a journal or your smartphone to record these answers. Don't filter them. Let it be a stream of consciousness. No one will see these—you can shred the pages afterward if you want, although I suggest keeping them so you can look back in three months to see how far you've progressed! While you can reexamine all of the memories that you write down, I've never found this to be necessary. Once the core memories are reinterpreted and released, the other memories lose their relevance and emotional charge. Write down every memory you have in response to the following question for your archetype:

Nurturer—When have you felt emotionally neglected?

Wonder Woman—When have you felt excluded or not fully accepted?

Femme Fatale—When have you felt less than because of the way you looked?

Ethereal—When have you felt alone in this world?

The responses I hear most frequently include feeling neglected by family members struggling with illness, addiction, or alcoholism; not fitting in at school because of your clothes; having less money than your school friends; being teased about a physical feature; a parent obsessed with their own looks; humiliation in front of the class; and a parent not supporting their child's passion.

If none of the questions above provokes any emotions, could being in denial be a way to make yourself feel more acceptable? Push yourself to look a little deeper.

THE EMOTION

What emotion do these memories evoke? (It's most often shame, sadness, or disappointment.)

_____

_____

_____

Which two memories are the most emotionally upsetting for you? Circle these. These are your core memories.

_____

_____

_____

THE JUDGMENT

What judgment are you attaching to these memories?

_____

_____

_____

The core memories have a judgment attached to them. There's an assumption that says, "It's not okay to——(insert word)" (e.g., be overweight, be poor, get things wrong, be alone, be emotional, wear the wrong clothes).

THE PROTECTIVE PATTERNS

Now take the time to reflect on how these judgments are affecting your behavior. Answer each of these questions in turn, regardless of your archetype.

1. What behaviors have you put in place to shield yourself from that unpleasant emotion?

    _____

    _____

    _____

2. What do you do (or not do) in an effort to get people to like, accept, and value you?

    _____

    _____

    _____

3. Do these patterns show up in your relationship with food?

_____

_____

_____

Take your time to work through these questions, and don't move on to the next one until you have answered the previous one. Your core memories will evoke powerful feelings within you that may surprise you at first, especially if you haven't thought about these memories in a long time. Don't let this upset you. Once you recognize the influence of the past, you can consciously start to dismantle your behavioral patterns.

CHAPTER 17

Reinterpret Your Past

———

Now that you have Recognized your core memory, it's time to Reinterpret it so you can let go of the misguided assumptions and beliefs that have stealthily influenced your behaviors. When these memories were formed, you were too young to process them correctly. But now that you have the benefit of hindsight and a better understanding of the forces that shaped your sense of self-worth, you can learn to look at these memories more rationally. This will free you from the emotions attached to those memories and help you discard the adaptive but ultimately self-sabotaging behaviors.

One of my core memories occurred when I was sixteen. I was having lunch at a café with my mother; younger sister, Carly; and best friend, Shae. Shae was a swimwear model who looked like a cross between Angelina Jolie and Elle Macpherson. My sister looked like a cooler, less curvaceous version of Barbie. They each weighed about 110 pounds, as did my mother, and none of them had ever dieted. I, on the other hand, had been on a diet since I was twelve.

When the owner of the restaurant came over to say hello to my mother, she proudly said she was with her two daughters. The owner said, "These two," pointing to Carly and Shae. My mother corrected him and everyone at the table laughed at his mistake—except me. In my mind I had been ostracized, deemed not attractive (or skinny) enough to be my own mother's daughter. This man's innocent mistake would leave a wound so jagged that it scarred me for years to come.

For two decades I would believe that my smeary lens of unattractiveness had interpreted that event correctly. But years later, I told this story to a friend who brushed it off and said, "Oh, you probably just dressed differently than the others." In that moment, I saw it all—the tape on rewind, the poison I had swallowed, the daggers that had cut away at my self-worth. All lies! The man's error had nothing to do with how attractive I was; it was simply pattern recognition, and I was the outlier. I looked like Snow White with jet black hair, wearing a pretty dress with ruby red lipstick, while the other three women were bronzed beachside blondes wearing jeans and tank tops, an outfit reminiscent of *Sports Illustrated* swimsuit models. It was like dropping a nun into the middle of the Playboy mansion. Our clothing choices couldn't have been more different!

Once I got over the shock of realizing how distorted my interpretation of this incident had been, I called my mother. Did she remember the event in question? Of course she didn't. Our memories encode best when we're fully present in the moment, and nothing makes you present like a charged emotion. I harbored the emotion of shame; she didn't. She reassured me that she had always thought I was attractive, words that revived my self-worth like an oxygen mask resuscitates a hyperventilating patient. Seeing this episode without my filter of unattractiveness was the third R—Reinterpretation.

Memories shape who we are for better and for worse. They allow us to learn from our mistakes and avoid situations that we know are dangerous. But they can also root us too firmly to the past as we spend our lives behaving in ways that protect us from a threat that doesn't exist. They are like blinders, keeping us too myopically focused on one thing while preventing us from seeing the whole picture.

The incidents that defined me as a woman were not tragic events but minor ones—like not being identified as my mother's daughter—that I'd misinterpreted to be more meaningful—and damning—than they were. Only by reexamining them under a different light—one brightened by compassion and empathy rather than shame—was I finally able to see how mistaken I'd been and the unnecessary pain I had caused myself.

No matter how disturbing or trifling the memory may be, reinterpreting it offers you a chance to heal. When you're attached to the memory, seeing beyond your filter can be near impossible. You can get caught up in thinking, "Of course it's true! It happened! I was there!" Indeed, the incident did happen, and there's no way to change it, but just as there are photographic filters that can alter how you view an image, your mind has thousands of filters to change how you view a memory.

One day, my normally mild-mannered client Mia went into a rage and threw a chair across the room after receiving a text from her mother. Her repressed anger had bubbled to the surface, and she couldn't contain it any longer. "I feel like such a disappointment," she confided to me. To the outside observer, she was anything but: she had a successful business, happy marriage, strong friendships, and an active social life. But behind this lay a troubled relationship with her mother, who refused to accept Mia's husband, despite their ten-year marriage. Mia resented her mother and felt her mother's love was extended only when she played into her mother's requests.

I asked Mia to read me the text message that had triggered the explosive reaction. It said: "I'm disappointed that you didn't respond earlier to the wedding invitation from your cousin." To the outside observer, this reads as nothing more than her mother telling her (if somewhat critically) that she was disappointed about a very specific thing. To Mia, it read, "*You are a disappointment*"—a subtle difference but a significant distortion that was causing her immense pain.

When I pointed this out to Mia, she was startled by her misinterpretation. Had her mother actually called her a disappointment as a child or had she just misinterpreted this, too? In that moment, she saw how insidious her filter of disappointment had been. It had weaved its way into her work and marriage. When her clients requested changes, she took this to mean that *she* had messed up (and was therefore a disappointment), rather than that her clients had simply changed their preference. When her husband asked her to do something, she assumed she had somehow disappointed him. She should have thought of this before he asked.

I asked Mia to speak to her mother. Did she really think she was a disappointment, and had she ever? The answer was a resounding no. Mia's mother very much admired and loved her daughter (even if she thought she was tardy with her wedding invitation response). She had also grown to like Mia's husband even though, at the time of their marriage, she wasn't sure if he was going to be successful enough for Mia. This much-needed mother-daughter conversation helped heal years of pain as Mia finally saw the distorted lens she had been living life through.

When my client Elizabeth was struggling to lose weight despite following a clean diet and exercising four times a week, I asked her if there might be something emotional blocking the weight loss. Her body fat looked like a protective cushion, and I suspected she was shielding herself from some past upset. She pondered this, then replied, "This is so silly, but I have a really painful memory from my wedding. When I proudly told my best friend (and bridesmaid) that I had lost twenty pounds for the wedding, she said she didn't even notice, and then after the wedding she ghosted me. I was distraught for two years, and it's still upsetting for me to look at our wedding photos with her in them." I suggested to Elizabeth that perhaps she had linked losing weight to losing friends and this was an emotional (and protective) reason for her to keep the weight on. If she lost weight again, would she lose friends again? Consciously she knew this wasn't true, but her subconscious didn't.

To reinterpret the memory, I asked a little bit about her friend.

Elizabeth explained that the friend came from an unstable family environment with a father who was often unfaithful. I suggested that perhaps her friend hadn't ghosted her because she lost weight but rather because by getting married Elizabeth had formed her own stable family unit, the antithesis of what her friend was used to. Rather than share Elizabeth's happiness, the wedding had pointed out what her friend was painfully lacking in her own life. Elizabeth will never know if this is true or not, but the "truth" here is irrelevant. We were simply trying to remove the sting from this memory and her belief that she had done something wrong to cause it.

Like Elizabeth, not everyone has the opportunity to speak to the parties involved in the memory. If you do, be bold and ask for their perspective, no matter how intimidating it may seem. This is not a blame game; you're not accusing them of ruining your sense of self. You're trying to get a more complete picture so you can heal. If you don't have that option, make up the most fantastical story you can think of, one that will make you laugh, and see how silly the misinterpretation you imposed on the situation is. It doesn't matter whether the new interpretation is true or not, only that it helps you wipe away the filter of shame that says, "I'm flawed and can therefore be discarded."

I've had to reinterpret several of my own childhood memories. One of the more painful memories occurred when I was seven years old reading in front of the class. I had an accent, having arrived in Australia from New Zealand the year before, and couldn't articulate the difference between "Bill" the farmer and a bull. "Bill" sounded like "bull" with my accent. My teacher was persistent and I felt humiliated by her. It was impossible for me to pronounce "Bill" the way she wanted me to. After that experience, my distraught seven-year-old self decided that the best thing to do was to avoid reading (and speaking) to groups ever again! But this desire to withdraw was thwarted because public speaking was part of the school curriculum. Instead, I would experience a huge surge of anxiety before I spoke, as if I was reliving the class humiliation.

Like most of us, I wasn't aware that this anxiety was being triggered from my upsetting childhood memory, I simply assumed I was one of those many millions of people who also feared public speaking. However, once I connected the two, I had my aha moment. Public speaking was not fear inducing; it was just making me relive the humiliation I felt as a child. When I recognized this association, I was able to reinterpret it. Since I couldn't go back to my second-grade teacher, I decided that her persistence in correcting my pronunciation was her seeing my potential and wanting me to flourish in life. It's irrelevant if it's true or not but it was certainly better than my previous filter, which said, "My second-grade teacher was a bitch and she humiliated me."

I was then able to believe, with both my conscious and subconscious mind, that a mispronounced word doesn't mean you are wrong, and being wrong doesn't mean you'll be humiliated. Today, I have simply accepted that I will mispronounce a word (I have an Australian accent and live in the United States) and just laugh it off. My reinterpreted memory dissolved my anxiety around public speaking and I now relish the idea of speaking to large audiences.

EXERCISE

1. Take two of the core memories that you unearthed in the last chapter and reinterpret them using compassion and love. Ask yourself, "How can I look at this memory through a different lens?" Remember, the new interpretation doesn't need to be the truth—you're just changing the way you view the memory. If you're attached to your original interpretation of the memory, you might need the help of an imaginative friend to offer you some rose-colored glasses to soften the focus. Write down the memory and reinterpretation.

ORIGINAL MEMORY	REINTERPRETED MEMORY

2. How does this new perception make you feel? Are you more at ease? Do you feel less triggered by the memory?

_____

_____

_____

3. Forgive yourself for your misinterpretation and anyone else in this memory that upset you. They most likely didn't realize how strongly the event registered with you.

_____

_____

_____

If you'd like to reinterpret other memories that touch off a heightened emotional response, do so. I've found that once you reinterpret the core memories, the little ones lose their power even more quickly.

By reinterpreting these core memories, the shame of them melts away and you break the judgment that your self-worth was built upon. The protective patterns you have put in place to insulate you from experiencing that feeling again are no longer needed. The self-worth matrix cracks.

CHAPTER 18

Release Your Emotions

―――

Once you have Recognized and Reinterpreted your core memories, the emotional charge attached to the memory will lessen, bringing an immediate sense of relief. However, rarely does an intellectual understanding of a damaging memory completely dissolve the pain attached to it. Most often there are lingering emotions, almost as if your cells have stored that memory with that emotion. In psychophysiology, there's a well-known saying: "What the mind forgets, the body remembers." Freud famously said, "Unexpressed emotions will never die. They are buried alive and will come forth later in uglier ways."

You can't change the fact that past, painful events occurred, but you *can* change the body's physical response to events that trigger those memories and the negative emotions associated with them. This is the forth R, and it allows you to physically Release the hold your core memories have on you.

FEELING SAFE WITH YOUR MEMORIES

There are two types of fear responses: instinctive and learned. Instinctive fear occurs in a life-or-death situation, like an ax-wielding man coming after you on a dark night. Overhearing an offhand comment about your weight, having no friends, or being humiliated at work are not life-or-death situations, but if you attach a negative emotion to them, they can cause the same stress response. This is called "learned fear" because your mind has associated the negative experience with fear. This fear is stored in the amygdala, and whenever a similar situation arises, it will tap into the memory and initiate the preprogrammed "fight-flight-freeze" stress response, characterized by sweaty palms, an elevated heart rate, anxiety, panic, immobilization, and an upset stomach.

But just as you can learn to feel fear, you can also learn to feel safety. As with learned fear, learned safety is the result of learning to associate a particular stimulus (an event, person, place, or situation) with protection from harm. When Nobel laureate Eric Kandel and his research team created safety conditions for rodents that they had previously made frightened, there was a dramatic reduction in their fear. In one study, mice were forced to swim in a pool of water—a desperate situation for them. The safety-conditioned mice overcame their sense of hopelessness while the fear-conditioned mice panicked and became very distressed.[1]

The researchers also noticed that learned safety increased brain-derived neurotrophic factor, BDNF, which creates new neurons and connections. There was also less activity in the amygdala, where fear memories are formed. Learned safety also altered the genetic expression of dopamine and the neuropeptide system (groups of chemicals that influence emotion) in the amygdala.[2]

This research suggests that you can learn to feel safe with your core memory. Instead of viewing the circumstances of that memory as inherent stressors that trigger a negative emotion, you can learn to associate those circumstances with a neutral outcome. By doing this, you can rewire your brain in a similar way to reprocessing your memory with a safety filter. Your mind imprints the memory with safety, which in turn alters your physical and emotional responses to situations that trigger the memory. The effects of anxiety, depression, and stress become muted, just like they did with the safety-conditioned mice.

When the core memory no longer causes painful emotional and physical responses, your protective behaviors become obsolete. You don't need to say yes to everyone, stay in a depleting job, endure a bad relationship, or diminish your self-worth because someone made an offhand comment about you. The barriers that you created to protect yourself from the negative emotions associated with a painful memory can be dismantled because the protective armor is no longer needed.

CREATING SAFETY: THE TECHNIQUES— EFT AND YOGIC BREATH

The two safety modalities that I use in my practice are emotional freedom technique (EFT) and yogic breath practices from kundalini yoga. EFT was developed in the 1980s and uses the same energy points targeted by acupressure and acupuncture to release stored negative energy from the body. Kundalini yoga is an ancient yogic practice that is derived from raja yoga—the yoga for royalty. It combines meditation, mantras, breath, and music to enhance consciousness and improve mental control.

Both approaches require you to recall an upsetting memory, feel the emotion, and then release the emotion through a physical action—either tapping or breathing, respectively. Both will Release the residual emotional charge of the memory.

Emotional Freedom Technique

Frequently referred to as "tapping," EFT uses acupressure and acceptance therapy to invoke safety and dissolve the energetic disturbance of a memory. Acupressure uses the same pressure points and meridians as acupuncture, but instead of needles, it uses firm finger pressure. Acceptance therapy asks you to accept the situation without judgment or the impulse to act on thoughts and emotions.

Psychologist and EFT practitioner Dr. Mary Ayers describes EFT using a computer analogy: Imagine your memories, stored in the amygdala, as a file. EFT finds the file and gives it a name, then you tap the file while saying its name and opening it up. Focusing on the file (or memory) activates the mind and triggers the same "freeze" response in your body that you originally experienced when the memory was formed. Tapping while the file is open is like hitting the delete key to uninstall an old program, one that is outdated or flawed. When you replay the old experience in your mind, you find that it no longer triggers those old feelings. The memory is still there but without its physical and emotional response.

Research is also supporting this. In one study, EFT was so powerful that after just a *single* hour-long session, study participants reported a 50 percent reduction in their anxiety and depression.[3] There was also a 24 percent reduction in cortisol levels, with some participants experiencing a whopping 50 percent drop in cortisol. In comparison, there was no significant cortisol reduction in those who underwent an hour of psychotherapy. Similarly, veterans with post-traumatic stress disorder (PTSD) who underwent ten hour-long EFT sessions saw their PTSD score decrease by 50 percent. These gains were maintained six months later, even though no more EFT was given. The EFT also altered six of the genes involved in PTSD.[4]

The basic sequence of EFT involves locating an emotional upset and then tapping twelve meridian points in the body. Meridian points are located along the path through which energy—what the ancient Chinese referred to as "ch'i"—flows throughout the body. As you tap these merid-ian points, you concentrate on the problem at hand—in this case your core memory. As you do this, the tapping motion sends a signal to the body and rebalances the energy so that the emotion associated with it is released. Essentially you are creating a condition of safety that demon-strates to your body that there is no need to be afraid of the memory; it is not a threat that requires you to fight, fly, or freeze. This releases the emo-tional charge that previously directed your behavior so you are no longer wired to respond a particular way whenever the memory resurfaces.

Dr. Mary Ayers has created a video series for you to experience EFT. You'll find it at danajames.com.

Yogic Breathing—Kundalini Yoga

Breathing is so fundamental to life that it has a dual control system: un-conscious breathing through the autonomic nervous system and conscious breathing through the voluntary nervous system. A three-minute con-scious breath series will transform an angry, frustrated, or upset woman into a calm, graceful, feminine woman who likes herself again. It works faster than a glass of wine and doesn't come with the guilt-shame cycle that a doughnut does! Yet most of us live in unconscious breath, unaware of how powerful conscious breath is in changing our emotional state.

Rhythmic breath activates a part of the brain called the periaqueductal gray (PAG) area, which has the brain's richest concentration of opioid recep-tors. By regulating your breath with deep rhythmic breathing, quick breaths, or holding your breath, you alter how the neuropeptides communicate with the PAG. You can direct your breath to be calming or stimulating, or to reduce fear, depression, anxiety, irritation, and sadness.

Richard Brown, MD, a psychiatrist and assistant professor at Colum-bia University, performed a study in which participants learned a thirty-minute yogic breath series called Sudarshan Kriya for five days. Sudarshan Kriya is one of the kundalini kriyas, a special type of meditation where music, breath, movement, and meditation are all combined. In the experiment, the Sudarshan Kriya produced a significant reduction in anxiety in patients, including those who had failed to achieve results with cognitive behavioral therapy and mindfulness-based stress reduction (MBSR), the gold standard in anxiety treatment.[5]

Similarly, Helen Lavretsky, MD, a psychiatrist and professor at UCLA, conducted an eight-week study in which she compared the effects of a daily twelve-minute kundalini breath series called Kirtan Kriya with listening to relaxing music on the mental and cognitive state of people caring for a family member with dementia. More than 60 percent of the study participants in the Kirtan Kriya group saw a 50 percent reduction in depression. This reduction in their depression was more than twice that of the group that listened to relaxing music.[6] Kirtan Kriya is included in the Femme Fatale's kundalini kriyas (but it is suitable for all archetypes).

If you have an overactive mind, kundalini kriyas can help you more easily slip into a relaxed meditative state. Kundalini is now my preferred meditation practice as I find the results more instantaneous due to the incorporation of the breath. When women come into my practice, I start them on two simple yogic breath techniques derived from kundalini yoga—O-mouth breath and breath of fire—depending on what I believe they need. I use O-mouth breath as part of a kundalini exercise called "Fists of Anger." When I guided my client Simone through the three-minute Fists of Anger exercise, she was able to forgive the children who had traumatized her with racially motivated taunts as a child and even threatened to kill her because her skin was a different color. As tears rolled down her face she said, "They were just stupid kids. It wasn't me. It wasn't my fault." Fists of Anger is incredibly healing and is included in both the Wonder Woman and the Nurturer's kundalini series, though any archetype can use it. Guru Jagat, kundalini teacher and author of *Invincible Living*, and I have created a three-part kundalini series for each of the archetypes. You will find instructions on how to perform each kriya in Appendix B, as well as instructional videos at danajames.com.

Conscious breathing instantly moves the body away from the "fight-flight-freeze" response. Try it now. Inhale deeply through your nose for a count of five, hold the breath for a count of five, then breathe out through your nose for a count of five. I suspect you felt slightly calmer after just one conscious breath. Imagine what three minutes can do!

I apply these two release techniques differently. For releasing the core memories I use EFT, as it is so effective in creating a sense of safety around the stored memory. Conscious breath is excellent for releasing the smaller memories and helping to maintain the reduced emotional charge of the core memories. There are certainly other release techniques, but I know these two work quickly and are supported by the medical literature.

The practice of Recognizing, Reinterpreting, and Releasing your memories can be applied as often as you need. Once you resolve the core memories, you can use these tools to address any future stressors associated with those memories that arise.

CHAPTER 19

Rewire Your Brain

N ow that you have tools to cope with the hidden drivers of your decision-making process, you are well on your way toward healing yourself of self-sabotaging behaviors. You can see into your blind spots as you become much more self-aware and conscious of your actions.

But habits—the conditioned responses that Pavlov discovered with his drooling dog—also influence your behaviors. Fortunately, habits are less imprinted than your core memories, and many of them are just a coping mechanism for dealing with those memories. For instance, if you use eating as an activity to escape disappointment, frustration, or uncertainty, you'll find it easier to stop now that you've reinterpreted and released your core memories.

Because habit formation is a conscious process (i.e., you're aware of what you are doing), breaking habits is much easier than reprogramming your subconscious. You don't need to mine the mind for answers; you simply need to do something different from what you did yesterday. Once Pavlov stopped giving food to the dogs when he rang the bell, over time they stopped stop salivating at the sound. Their brains learned the bell was no longer associated with food and their conditioned response reversed. If a dog's brain can be deprogrammed, so can yours. Rewiring your brain to form new habits is the fifth R.

WHAT IS A HABIT?

Habits are created when you associate two things—a stimulus and a response—with each other and then repeat that response whenever you're presented with the stimulus. An example could be coming home from work (stimulus) and pouring yourself a glass of wine (response). Or walking past your coworker's desk (stimulus) and grabbing a handful of M&M's from her shared jar (response). The more you repeat the behavior, the more cemented the habit becomes because your brain remembers the association. Through repetition, you strengthen the synaptic connection, creating larger and stronger neural networks, just like muscles that are trained repeatedly at the gym.

The stronger the neural network, the more instinctual it is for you to do something. While this process is incredibly helpful for many day-to-day activities, like riding a bike, driving a car, remembering the route to work, and using your phone, it can also create less beneficial habits—like mindlessly eating M&M's, drinking wine automatically at the end of every day, and even a binge-purge response.

When you want to break a habit, your brain needs to create new synaptic connections and a new neural pathway. The brain doesn't want to have to create new brain cells if it doesn't have to. It also doesn't understand why you want to change your habitual patterns. If you've been eating cookies every night for the past two years, and one night you decide that you've had enough, your mind will try to outsmart you so you keep eating cookies. The brain doesn't judge which habits are good for you and which aren't; it simply follows the neural networks that have been created because that's what it's trained itself to do.

That means when you try to break a nonsupportive habit, you might hear voices that give you permission to stay stuck in it. CBT calls these voices "distorted thought patterns." If you're a nighttime eater looking to break that habit, the voices might sound like this:

- It's only a bite.
- I can start my diet tomorrow.
- I'm hungry.
- I won't be able to sleep unless I eat.
- I'm not *that* fat so it's okay for me to have a treat tonight.
- It's better than pizza.
- I'm never going to lose the weight so I may as well feel good now.
- It's not fair. Why can't I eat whatever I want?
- Screw it!
- I deserve it!

If you try to argue with or ignore these voices, they'll get louder. Instead, acknowledge them for what they are—a way for your brain to avoid having to create new brain cells—and shut down the conversation. If these thoughts enter your head, tell yourself, "I hear you, but you're not a commandment from God. You're a voice that makes me lose my integrity to myself and that makes me feel guilty afterward for not sticking to my word." With an adamant no, you end the conversation.

You may fear that unless you eat the food, the voice won't go away. I promise you it will. Only when you can't make up your mind will the voice continue to torment you. A firm decision—yes or no—will stop the voice. "Yes" depletes your integrity. "No" reclaims it. Sit with the discomfort that emerges when you say no. It passes. Just like other habits you've broken, you can break that nighttime cookie habit, too.

A QUICK WAY TO BREAK A HABIT

For those times when your "No" isn't as rock solid as it needs to be, I want you to have a quick and dirty trick to stop the habit in its tracks. It's not the ultimate solution, but it's effective. Try associating the habit with something grotesque. When you do so, your desire for it quickly diminishes and you will start rewiring your brain so you no longer crave it.

Choose a habit that you want to break—perhaps it's mindlessly eating those M&M's on your coworker's desk—and imagine that all of the candy has been slobbered on by the sniffly guy in accounting who is always sick. Eeww! If you want to stop pillaging the bread basket at a restaurant, imagine weevils crawling out of the bread and into your mouth. (It's like a horror film!) That nightly glass of wine is a lot less appealing when you imagine someone with athlete's foot stomping on the grapes! Yes, it's disgusting, but that's the point. And it doesn't need to be true; it just needs to stop you. The imagination is a powerful thing; use it to your advantage.

WHY ARE HABITS SO HARD TO BREAK?

When you feel like you can't break a habit, it's because you're getting a payoff from that habit. For Emily the payoff from her Friday-night pizza fest was connection. Emily feared that if she didn't eat the pizza, she'd lose her friends. Emily was able to break this habit when she realized she didn't need to eat pizza to achieve this connection and that the payoff of declining the pizza—sticking to her diet, keeping the weight off, and feeling more confident of her willpower—was bigger than the one she got from succumbing to temptation. Only when the benefit of stopping the habit exceeds the payoff does the habit lose its compulsion.

The payoff of your habits is not always obvious. Let's look at the Nurturer. She desperately wants to lose weight. Her wardrobe runs the gamut from size 2 to size 10, and the thought of going up another size is humiliating. Her doctor has warned her that she's prediabetic and she needs to vigilantly watch her sugar intake. There's a tremendous upside to skipping that morning muffin with her coffee, but she's also getting a payoff. She's got way too much to think about in the morning—kids to organize, dog to feed, clothes that don't fit, the commute—it's chaos. She can't possibly fit in another thing, like making a smoothie for herself for breakfast. Picking up a muffin is easy. Besides, her four-year-old hates the noise of the blender. The muffin is something she looks forward to, and the thought of skipping it feels like deprivation. She hates feeling deprived. She hates dieting, too. Scarfing down that muffin feels like a kind of rebellion. Given all of the odds stacked against it, is the smoothie going to win out? My bet is on the muffin.

Or what about Wonder Woman? She'd like to give up her nightly glass of red wine because it's interfering with her sleep, making her less focused, and she's put on ten pounds in the past year. To the outside observer, those facts should be enough motivation to cut back on the wine. But what if she's using the wine to wind down from the day and without it she's worried she'll snap at her two-year-old or not be able to relax because otherwise she can't stop thinking about the mountain of work waiting for her at the office the next day? Wonder Woman is getting a lot of hidden benefits from her habit besides a fruity bouquet.

But the wine and the muffin aren't actually the issue. They're decoys that distract from the real issues these women are facing. If they want to break these habits, they need to look at the reasons they formed in the first place and figure out a new habit that provides the same payoff without all the guilt and shame. For the Nurturer, this may mean giving herself some "me" time before she opens the door to the morning chaos. For Wonder Woman, this may mean leaving the office earlier and not responding to emails after seven p.m. These aren't easy tasks when these women value themselves on being there for others or making sure that no work falls through the cracks. But once the memories that forged your archetype's

dominance have been reinterpreted and released, you'll find it much easier to break these habits because the precarious foundation upon which
your archetype derives her self-worth has been dismantled. Remember,
it's not knowledge that breaks a pattern; it's the experience of actually
changing the habit that does.

FIND A REPLACEMENT HABIT

Doing nothing at the time you normally engage in your habit can feel like
purgatory. You'll have all this free time to think about your habit, whether
it's eating cookies or stalking an ex on social media, and you'll often crack
because the space is so unfamiliar and uncomfortable to you. Instead,
find something that brings you pleasure. Far too many women live a life
devoid of pleasure, often because it's perceived as a luxury. It's not. It's a
core component of being human and feeling alive. When you create a
habit that is truly pleasurable, the new payoff is a life full of richness
and joy.

In the next chapter, we'll explore this more, but for now, think about
the payoff you are getting from your habit and what alternative behavior
might result in the same benefit. For instance, the Wonder Woman is
clutching her nightly glass of wine because it gives her permission to
switch off. Once she's had half a glass of wine, she can't go back to her
emails under the haze of alcohol. What could she do instead? First, she
can remind herself that she has permission to relax because she needs to
recharge. She doesn't need a glass of wine to give her an excuse. She can
then make herself a cup of Wonder Woman tea and curl up next to her
husband on the sofa while they talk and connect. If she's single, she can
slip into a silk robe, sip her tea, and read an engrossing book for an hour
instead.

EXERCISE

When you identify a habit that you'd like to break, ask yourself these questions:

1.   What's the hidden payoff you are currently getting from this habit?

_____

_____

_____

2.   What's the benefit of *not* engaging in the habit? Use emotions to describe this since emotions drive our behavior (e.g., to feel alive, more confident, proud).

_____

_____

_____

3.   What's a new pleasurable habit that you could cultivate instead?

_____

_____

_____

4.   When will you replace the old habit with the new habit?

_____

_____

_____

5.   What will thwart this effort, and why? How can you change this?

_____

_____

_____

The more consciously you consider the habits you want to break, the more consistently you'll be able to Rewire your brain to form new habits. The result is not just an end to unproductive behaviors but the beginning of becoming a more empowered woman who has integrity to herself.

CHAPTER 20

Revive Your Sense of Self

═══

The first five Rs helped you shed the out-of-balance behaviors of your archetype, but in order to reach your crown, you need to incorporate the best qualities of all the *other* archetypes into your life. Tapping into your inner Nurturer, Wonder Woman, Femme Fatale, and Ethereal will help you reconnect with your true feminine self. If you're a Nurturer who has always envied the Ethereal's free spiritedness, or if you're a Wonder Woman who wants to connect with her sensual Femme Fatale, or if you simply want to expand your life to become more enriching and fulfilling, the sixth R—Revive—will help you do all of this and more.

I call this step Revive because you already have the qualities of each archetype within you but because of your childhood imprints, cultural beliefs, and protective behaviors, you haven't always cultivated these positive attributes. Now it's time to Revive them.

YOUR FULFILLMENT LIST

The first step toward reviving yourself and reconnecting with the other archetypes is to create opportunities for pleasure in your life. By engaging in activities that feel enjoyable, you automatically bring out your feminine energies to reconnect with your hidden archetypes. Pleasure isn't something you need to *earn*; rather, it's critical to keeping you vitalized and engaged in life. Without it, you'll dry up and become brittle and resentful.

Engaging in activities that feel pleasurable enables you to live a more fulfilling life. Fulfillment stems from connection—with others, yourself, the earth, and to a purpose beyond yourself. When you are truly fulfilled, you are not worried about the expectations of the outside world. You are free to enjoy life.

Start thinking about the activities that you enjoy. This may be something as simple as sipping a cup of organic coffee first thing in the morning, or taking a walk in the park on a sunny spring afternoon. Or it can be something more extravagant like a two-week trip to Bali to commune with nature and your spiritual self. Assume money isn't a constraint. You'll find that many of life's most fulfilling things don't cost much money.

Be very granular. Include authors you like to read, movement classes you enjoy, or routines that bring balance and harmony to your life. Leave alcohol and pleasure foods off the list for now. I want you to find activities outside the sensations of food. But otherwise, don't limit yourself. If you love to paint but you haven't picked up a brush in twenty years, that's okay—if it still brings you joy, add it to the list.

Once you've listed at least thirty things, sort them by frequency— things you can do daily, monthly, seasonally, and annually. When I did this for myself, I wrote "swimming in the Mediterranean" on the annual list. While I'd love to do that daily, it won't happen while I live in the United States, but it did direct my summer vacation to Italy that year. It was worth investing money in something that truly made me feel joyful.

You should end up with more daily activities than monthly, seasonal, or annual ones because the greater the pool of daily activities, the more options you have for adding daily fulfillment to your life. You probably won't do each thing every day, but the idea is to think of things you *can* do often because they don't require much effort or advance planning. Even if the only thing you do on a given day is to meditate for ten minutes or read a bedtime story to your kids, your life is going to feel good because you've done at least one thing that makes you feel joyful. If you do more, then you've added more richness to your life.

Fulfillment List

DAILY	MONTHLY	SEASONALLY	ANNUALLY

Remember that fulfillment is about connection to yourself, others, the earth, and a higher purpose. Let that guide you if you get stuck. Sometimes, you've just forgotten what you like. If you need some inspiration, take a look at the lists of activities for each archetype below. I want you to become a complete woman, and one way to do that is by exploring the elements of yourself that you might not have paid attention to for a while.

In addition to being pleasurable in their own right, the activities on this fulfillment list can also be useful when you want to form replacement habits. If you've been getting hidden rewards from your eating habits, think about how these other activities may provide the same—or even greater—benefit. When I was breaking my sugar compulsion, I'd often watch a TED Talk (or three) until the urge subsided. It was a transitional fix while I worked on the underlying cause of the cravings, and it provided the same reward—a way to switch off—with none of the post-eating shame.

Archetype Activities List

NURTURER Positive Traits: compassion, loyalty, warmth

ACTIVITIES:

Cooking dinner with friends
Reading a bedtime story to or playing with your kids
Laughing with family or friends
Buying flowers for yourself
Shopping at the farmers market
Volunteering at a local soup kitchen or homeless shelter

WONDER WOMAN Positive Traits: dignity, drive, intellect

ACTIVITIES:

Taking a foreign language class
Reading a thought-provoking article or book
Watching TED Talks or listening to podcasts
Taking an exercise class
Visiting a museum

FEMME FATALE Positive Traits: sensuality, playfulness, fun

ACTIVITIES:

Date night with your partner
Taking photographs
Dancing
Reading a juicy novel
Taking a luxurious bath
Making love to your partner
Getting a massage

ETHEREAL Positive Traits: creativity, intuition, imagination

ACTIVITIES:

Morning meditation
Taking a yoga class
Painting
Reading spiritual books
Burning incense, candles, or essential oils
Hiking in the woods
Swimming in the ocean

Don't think of the items on your Fulfillment List as other things you *need* to do. It's about knowing what you *like* to do. For a life filled with more richness, try incorporating two things from the list into your routine every day and planning at least one of the less-regular activities—like a vacation—for sometime in the near future. Engaging in activities from your Fulfillment List is how you're supposed to live. These aren't monetary riches but life's riches.

THE BEAUTY OF CONNECTION

While every woman's Fulfillment List will look different, there is one thing that every women needs to include if they want to live a fulfilling life and ascend to their crown: connection. Our biology is hardwired for human connection (after all, it takes at least two people to continue the survival of our species). According to Candace Pert, PhD, who discovered the first opioid receptor in the brain, human connection is why we produce the body's neurochemicals. Pert calls these chemicals "molecules of emotion." She states that there are more than 250 neuropeptides that act as molecules of emotions. When you connect deeply with someone, serotonin, dopamine, oxytocin, and hundreds of other neuropeptides have the potential to be released and positively alter how you feel. This is part of the reason food and antidepressants are poor surrogates for intimate connection. They only target one or two individual neurotransmitters, not the hundreds of other neuropeptides.

Steve Cole, a genomic researcher at the University of California, Los Angeles, observed that lonely people and social people had a different gene expression in 209 genes, many of which affected the immune system.[1] According to Cole, "Loneliness really is one of the most threatening experiences we can have."[2] If loneliness damages the immune system, then it becomes a risk factor for depression, anxiety, heart disease, dementia, obesity, autoimmune conditions, and cancer—all diseases that are influenced by inflammation triggered by the immune response.

Similarly, when women with binge-eating tendencies perceive themselves to be socially isolated, their binge eating increases. Women who have recovered from an eating disorder say their recovery was largely influenced by a deeper connection with themselves and others.[3] Recovery from other addictions, such as alcohol and recreational drugs, is also bolstered by connection. Community is part of the reason Alcoholics Anonymous can be so effective.

It's not just a matter of finding a mate to make you feel connected. Germaine Greer, feminist and author of *The Female Eunuch*, said, "Many a housewife staring at the back of her husband's newspaper, or listening to his breathing in bed is lonelier than any spinster in a rented room." Connection is more than the presence of another person. It's feeling like you belong and are valued. It's the ability to give and receive affection. Connection feels warm and emotionally safe.

Being in the company of others in a group fitness class, a group meditation, or a yoga class will also elevate the molecules of emotion. There's a bonding experience that takes place that doesn't happen when you're alone. It's why boutique group fitness classes took off and why meditating in a group produces a more heightened sense of awareness than when you are on your own. It's why more spiritually aligned women are hosting goddess and moon circles or are going to church. It's why book clubs were created. It's why tea salons came into existence. It's why the Coliseum was erected. It's why social media was invented. It's about connection. Pleasure is the by-product.

How do you create an intimate and heartwarming connection? Be open and honest. Get curious about other people. Be vulnerable. Make the connection pure. Purity happens when you've salved your own childhood wounds with forgiveness and you've healed the scars of your past with a new interpretation.

My hope is that this book has helped you do just that and that you continue to draw inspiration from it as you seek more fulfillment in your life. Connection is so fundamental for our feminine essence that I've curated interviews from well-known women who are at their crown, as well as videos for recipes, kundalini, EFT, meditation, and making teas. These are available at danajames.com. Consider this a place to go for inspiration and ideas as you begin your journey on the Archetype Model.

PARTING WORDS

Every woman deserves this information, and it's my privilege to share it with you. I am deeply proud of the Archetype Model. I hope you have taken the steps toward reaching your crown and are inspired enough to share the archetype lifestyle with other women (and men—they'll benefit too!). As we understand ourselves better and shed the insecurities that hold us back, we can connect on a deeper level. We become more open, more loving, and more united. We become the fabric of the new feminine way of thinking, feeling, and being, in a society that desperately needs new feminine role models. I hope you become one, and I trust you will.

Food Types

Vegetables

CRUCIFEROUS

Bok choy
Broccoli
Broccoli rabe
Brussels sprouts
Cabbage
Cauliflower
Collard greens
Kale
Kohlrabi
Mustard greens
Spinach
Swiss chard
Watercress

GREEN LEAFY

Arugula
Butter lettuce
Cress
Dandelion greens
Escarole
Frisée
Gem lettuce
Mixed greens
Romaine

GREEN

Artichoke
Asparagus
Celery
Cucumber
Endive
Green beans
Okra
Peas
Snow peas
Sugar snap peas
Zucchini

RED

Radicchio
Radish
Red beets
Red bell peppers
Red onion
Tomatoes

ORANGE

Carrots
Orange bell peppers

YELLOW

Golden beets
Sweet corn
Yellow bell peppers
Yellow tomatoes

PURPLE

Eggplant
Purple cabbage
Purple carrots
Purple-sprouting
broccoli

WHITE

Celeriac
Fennel
Garlic
Jicama
Leeks
Onions
Ramps
Scallions
Shallots
Sunchokes

BROWN

Mushrooms
(shiitake,
maitake, button,
crimini, oyster,
portobello)

Fruit

GREEN

Green apples
Honeydew melon
Kiwifruit
Limes
Pears

RED

Cherries
Guava
Pink and red
grapefruit
Pomegranate
Raspberries
Red apples
Rhubarb
Strawberries
Watermelon

ORANGE

Apricots
Cantaloupe
Clementines
Gooseberries
Mango
Nectarines
Oranges
Papaya
Peaches
Persimmons
Tangerines

YELLOW

Golden kiwifruit
Grapefruit
Lemons
Passionfruit
Pineapple
Yellow
watermelon

PURPLE

Acai
Blackberries
Blueberries
Boysenberries
Dates
Figs
Plums
Prunes
Purple grapes

Complex Carbohydrates

GRAINS

Amaranth
Brown rice
Buckwheat
Millet
Quinoa
Wild rice

LEGUMES

Black beans
Cannellini beans
Chickpeas
Edamame
Flageolet beans
Lentils (orange,
green, black)
Pinto beans
Red kidney beans

STARCHY VEGETABLES

Parsnips
Potatoes (white, red, and purple)
Pumpkin
Sweet potatoes
Turnips
Winter squash
Yams

Protein

OILY FISH

Arctic Char
Anchovies
Black cod
Halibut
Herring
Mackerel
Sardines
Trout
Tuna
Wild salmon

WHITEFISH

Cod
Dover Sole
Haddock
Hake
Flounder
Grey sole
Lemon sole
Mahi mahi
Monkfish

Perch
Red snapper
Skate
Sea bass
Sea bream
Tilapia
Whiting

SEAFOOD

Calamari
Clams
Crab
Lobster
Mussels
Octopus
Oysters
Scallops
Shrimp

POULTRY

Organic chicken
Organic duck
Organic turkey

RED MEAT

Grass-fed beef
Grass-fed bison
Grass-fed lamb
Grass-fed pork
Grass-fed veal
Grass-fed venison

PROTEIN POWDER

Collagen protein
powder

Hemp protein
powder
Pea protein
powder
Rice protein
powder

Fats

NUTS (RAW ONLY)

Almonds
Brazil nuts
Cashews
Chestnuts
Coconuts
Hazelnuts
Macadamia
Pecans
Pine nuts
Pistachios
Walnuts

SEEDS (RAW ONLY)

Chia
Flax
Hemp
Pumpkin
Sesame
Sunflower

OILS

Avocado oil

Coconut oil

Extra-virgin olive oil

Hemp seed oil

Macadamia oil

Walnut oil

VEGETABLES

Avocado

Olives

Herbs and Spices

FRESH

Basil

Chives

Cilantro

Oregano

Parsley

Rosemary

Thyme

DRIED

Cinnamon

Coriander powder

Cumin

Curry powder

Fennel seeds

Fenugreek

Mustard seeds

Nutmeg

Paprika

Pepper

Saffron

Sea salt

Star anise

Turmeric

Vanilla bean

Super Foods

Aloe vera juice

Barley grass

Cacao

Chlorophyll

Rose water

Spirulina

Wheatgrass

Kundalini Kriyas for Each Archetype

As a reminder, videos for these kriyas can be found at danajames.com.

NURTURER

1. Cat and Cow—2 minutes

Come onto your hands and knees in a tabletop position. Your hands are shoulder-width apart with your fingers pointing forward. The knees are directly below the hips. Close your eyes and begin to breathe deeply. As you inhale, tilt the pelvis forward, arching the spine down and stretching the head and neck back. When you exhale, tilt the pelvis up, arching the spine toward the ceiling and bringing the chin to the chest.

2. Fists of Anger—3 minutes

Sit cross-legged with your spine straight. Focus your mind on anything and everything that makes you angry. Continue to bring up these anger points throughout the meditation. Make an "O" shape with your mouth and begin to breathe deeply and rhythmically. As you breathe, touch each thumb to the base of the pinky finger on the same hand. Close the rest of the fingers over the thumbs to form fists. Raise the arms and begin a backstroke-type movement over the head, alternating each side (right/left) as you swing up, over, and back around again. As you continue, increase the movement of the arms and breath. This helps release stored emotions in the body like anger and frustration. To end, interlock your fingers on both hands, stretch the arms up overhead, palms facing up, and inhale deeply through the O-mouth. Picture yourself surrounded in white, healing light. Exhale out the O-mouth.

3. Sat Kriya—11 minutes

Tuck your knees under your body so you can sit on your heels. Use a blanket or block under your seat for support, if needed. With your spine straight, extend your arms overhead, elbows squeezing your ears, and interlace all fingers except your index fingers. Extend your index fingers toward the sky and press the finger pads together. Cross the left thumb over the right one. Keep this position throughout the meditation. With your eyes slightly open, focus on the tip of your nose. As you inhale, pull the breath to the spine and chant SAT! On the exhale, relax the belly and chant NAM, which should sound like a sigh. To end, inhale as you squeeze all your muscles from seat to shoulders and relax everything as you exhale.

WONDER WOMAN

1. Sufi Grinds—2 minutes

Sit cross-legged with the spine straight, eyes closed, and your hands on your knees. Move the body through large circles, keeping the head up and rotating from the hips. Inhale through the nose as you circle forward and exhale through the nose as you circle back. Do this for one minute and then reverse direction for one more minute.

2. Fists of Anger—3 minutes

See Nurturer

3. Cross-hearted Kirtan Meditation—11 minutes

Sit cross-legged with the spine straight and eyes focused on the tip of your nose. Cross your forearms below the wrist and hold them in front of the chest with the arms out slightly. Palms are faceup and slightly turned toward the chest. Practice relaxed breathing as you chant the mantra SA TA NA MA. Chant each syllable for one second as you touch your thumbs to each finger, starting with the index finger on SA and ending with the pinky finger on MA. Continue this throughout the meditation. To end, inhale and hold the breath for three seconds, focusing the eyes upward. Exhale and return to normal breathing.

FEMME FATALE

1. Sufi Grinds—2 minutes

See Wonder Woman

2. Sat Kriya—3 minutes

See Nurturer

3. Kirtan Kriya—12 minutes

Sit cross-legged with the spine straight and your focus at the brow point. Straighten the elbows and balance the backs of your hands on the top of each thigh. Chant the mantra SA TA NA MA. Chant each syllable for one second as you touch your thumbs to each finger, starting with the index finger on SA and ending with the pinky finger on MA. Continue this throughout the meditation. Begin the kriya in a normal voice for two minutes, then whisper for two minutes, then silently for four minutes. Then come back to a whisper for two minutes, then a normal voice for two minutes. To end, stretch the arms overhead and spread the fingers wide, shaking them out and circulating the energy for one minute. Inhale and exhale three times. Relax.

ETHEREAL

1. Spine Flex—2 minutes

Sit cross-legged with the spine straight and hold on to your ankles with your hands. Keep the eyes softly focused and engage in normal deep breathing. As you inhale, flex the spine forward, keeping your shoulders relaxed and head straight, and feel the energy go down the spine. As you exhale, round the spine back and feel the energy come back up the spine to the third eye. Chant silently "SAT" as you inhale and "NAM" as you exhale.

2. Sat Kriya—3 minutes

See Femme Fatale

3. Prosperity meditation—11 minutes

Sit cross-legged with the spine straight. Eyes are slightly open, staring at the tip of the nose. Elbows are by your sides and forearms are at a forty-five-degree angle with the hands at the level of the throat. Start with the palms facing down. Strike the sides of the hands together so the sides of the index fingers touch and the thumbs cross below the hands, with the right thumb under the left. Turn the palms up so the pinky fingers and the base of the palms touch. It looks like you're creating a box in the air. Breathe deeply, and chant HAR (sounds like "hu-duh") for the entire eleven minutes, striking your hands together, palms up and palms down.

Resources

─────

These are some of the highest quality supplements and brands that I trust and use with my clients in my clinical practice. Most of these supplements are available online but some are only available through a health-care practitioner. For your convenience, I have packaged the archetype supplements into an archetype kit and these are available at danajames.com.

ORGANIC PLANT PROTEIN

Dana James Beatifuel Plant Protein—danajames.com
Nue & Co Plant Protein + Gut Food—thenueco.com
The Super Elixir Nourishing Protein—welleco.com

NUTRITIONAL SUPPLEMENTS

Supplement Packs

Archetype Alchemy by Dana James—danajames.com
Archetype Adrenal Tonic—danajames.com

Probiotics

Klaire Labs Ther Biotic—klairelabs.com
Dr Ohhira's Professional Probiotics—drohhiraprobiotics.com
Xymogen ProbioMax—xymogen.com (available only to healthcare practitioners; use referral code JAMESDA to access)

Glucose regulating supplement

Designs for Health Metabolic Synergy—designsforhealth.com
Xymogen MedCaps IS—xymogen.com (available to healthcare practitioners; use referral code JAMESDA to access)

B Complex

Vital Nutrients B Complex—vitalnutrients.net

Vitamin C

Designs for Health C + Bio Fizz—designsforhealth.com
Perque Potent C Guard—perque.com
Vital Nutrients Vitamin C + Bioflavonoids—vitalnutrients.net

Magnesium

Klaire Labs Magnesium Citrate—klairelabs.com

Xymogen Magnesium Citrate—xymogen.com (only available to healthcare practitioners; use referral code JAMESDA to access)
Vital Nutrients Magnesium Glycinate/Malate—vitalnutrients.net

Phosphatidylserine

Integrative Therapeutics Cortisol Manager—integrativepro.com
NuMedica Phosphytidylserine—numedica.com
Xymogen NeuroActives BrainSustain—xymogen.com (available only to healthcare practitioners; use referral code JAMESDA to access)

5-HTP

Designs for Health 5-HTP Synergy—designsforhealth.com
Xymogen 5-HTP CR—xymogen.com (available only to healthcare practitioners; use referral code JAMESDA to access)

Thyroid Supplement

Young Living Thyromin—youngliving.com
Xymogen T-150—xymogen.com (available only to healthcare practitioners; use referral code JAMESDA to access)

Digestive Enzyme

Enzyme Science Critical Digestion—enzyscience.com

Omega-3 supplement

Xymogen Omega Pure—xymogen.com (available only to healthcare practitioners; use referral code JAMESDA to access)
Nordic Naturals Ultimate Omega—nordicnaturals.com

L-Carnitine

DFH Carnitine Tartrate—designsforhealth.com

DIM

Xymogen Hormone Protect—xymogen.com (available only to healthcare practitioners; use referral code JAMESDA to access)
Designs for Health DIM-Avail—designsforhealth.com

Candida Control

Enzyme Science Candida Control—enzyscience.com

Organic Aloe Vera Juice

Lily of the Desert Aloe Vera Juice—lilyofthedesert.com
Lakewood Organic Whole Leaf Aloe Juice—lakewoodjuices.com

ORGANIC HERBS

Banyan Botanicals—banyanbotanicals.com

Ashwaganda root
Rhodiola

Sun Potion—sunpotion.com

Ashwaganda root
Rhodiola
Cordyceps

ORGANIC TEA SUPPLIES

Tea Spot—teaspot.com
Bulk Apothecary—bulkapothecary.com
Zackwoods Herbs—zackwoodsherbs.com

WITH GRATITUDE

This book was years in the making. It was a constant process of refining and reshaping before it evolved into its current form. I have had many guides along the way.

First and foremost, thank you to my clients. Your trust was essential. You shed the countless tears that helped uncover the emotional reasons for your struggles with food. You let me be your "therapist" when you thought you were coming in for a food plan. You were vulnerable and honest and it was through your stories that I finally saw the link between self-worth and food.

Kim Hekimian at Columbia University, I cannot thank you enough for allowing me to explore shame and obesity. Your insight and persistent questions helped create this model that was so indirect that most people couldn't see the links. Thank you for believing in this noble cause and sharing research when it emerged.

Christine Arylo, you taught me the feminine way and without our exploration into female mythology I may not have found the archetypes. Thank you for helping me see my own unconscious patterns even when I resisted and wanted to give up. Johanna Carroll, your feminine and wise woman guidance was essential. It was your insistence that I discover the chakra imbalance in the archetypes that helped make this model more complete. Your creative insight on titles time and time again was invaluable.

Coleen O'Shea, my literary agent, thank you for seeing my potential and for ushering this book into the hands of publishers. Becky Cabaza, thank you for pulling together the proposal for this book. Without your expertise, this idea may not have ever made it to print. Jacquie Chamberlain for her assistance with creating the recipes for this book. My free-spiritedness in the kitchen does not translate well to a constructed set of directions. Every reader also thanks you!

Brooke Carey, my fearless editor, without you, there would be no book. Or not a great one. You refined, edited, and made this book what it is today.

Thank you, thank you for being my Wonder Woman match and replicating my voice through the words on the pages of this book. Pam Krauss, thank you for making this book a far, far better book. Your astute eye simplified the archetype model. Without your vision for what it could be, it would have been a messy book. Thank you to the rest of the team at Avery/Penguin for believing in this book and getting it onto bookshelves—online and offline.

To the pioneers whose work inspired me: Mark Hyman, Frank Lipman, Kelly Brogan, Louise Hay, Marianne Williamson, Brené Brown, Gabby Bernstein, Christiane Northrup, Lissa Rankin, Bruce Lipton, Deepak Chopra, Joseph Campbell, Gloria Steinem, and Caroline Myss. If it wasn't for your work leading the way, I wouldn't have seen the mind-body connection that now is as clear as a sparkling diamond.

Thank you to my parents for being open and honest when I asked questions about my own childhood. You helped make more sense of what seemed painful and incongruent. I was the guinea pig for my own model.

Nadya Andreeva and Lisa Merkle, your unconditional friendship makes everything seem brighter. Thank god you are in my life. And for all of my girlfriends who listened and read chapters and gave their invaluable feedback.

Alexandra Defacio for your purity, your spiritual guidance, and a bosom to rest in. You are my Nurturer who taught me so much about myself.

Clement Kwan, you simply make my life better. You are showing me how to love, how to receive help, and how to express my own vulnerabilities. Without you and your daring support, this book wouldn't make it into the hands of the many, many women who need it.

And last, to all the women I have had conversations with; even if I can't name you, your feelings are echoed in this book. This is a book that explores a woman's mind and you shared your stories with me. I look forward to talking more now that this book has been created.

NOTES

CHAPTER 2: THE NURTURER

1   K. M. Gavin, E. E. Cooper, and R. C. Hickner. "Estrogen receptor protein content is different in abdominal than gluteal subcutaneous adipose tissue of overweight-to-obese premenopausal women." *Metabolism* 62, no. 8 (2013): 1180–88.

2   B. F. Palmer and D. J. Clegg. "The sexual dimorphism of obesity." *Mol Cell Endicronal* 402 (2015): 113–119.

3   S. R. Dube, D. Fairweather, W. S. Pearson, V. J. Felitti, R. F. Anda, and J. B. Croft. "Cumulative childhood stress and autoimmune diseases in adults." *Psychosomatic Medicine* 71, no. 2 (2009): 243–50.

4   T. Opala, P. Rzymski, I. Pischel, M. Wilczak, and J. Wozniak. "Efficacy of 12 weeks supplementation of a botanical extract-based weight loss formula on body weight, body composition and blood chemistry in healthy, overweight subjects—a randomised double-blind placebo-controlled clinical trial." *European Journal of Medical Research* 11, no. 8 (2006): 343–50.

5   A. P. Tardivo, J. Nahas-Neto, C. L. Orsatti, F. B. Dias, P. F. Poloni, E. B. Schmitt, and E. A. Nahas. "Effects of omega-3 on metabolic markers in postmenopausal women with metabolic syndrome." *Climacteric* 18, no. 2 (2015): 290–98.

6   M. Pooyandjoo, M. Nouhi, S. Shab-Bidar, K. Djafarian, and A. Olyaeemanesh. "The effect of (L-)carnitine on weight loss in adults: a systematic review and meta-analysis of randomized controlled trials." *Obesity Reviews* 17, no. 10 (2016): 970–76.

7   F. Brouns and G. J. van der Vusse. "Utilization of lipids during exercise in human subjects: metabolic and dietary constraints." *British Journal of Nutrition* 79, no. 2 (1998): 117–28.

8   Rajoria, S., R. Suriano, P. S. Parmar, Y. L. Wilson, U. Megwalu, A. Moscatello, H. L. Bradlow, D. W. Sepkovic, J. Geliebter, S. P. Schantz, and R. K. Tiwari (2011). "3,3'-diindolylmethane modulates estrogen metabolism in patients with thyroid proliferative disease: a pilot study." *Thyroid* 21(3): 299–304.

CHAPTER 3: THE WONDER WOMAN

1   D. Spar. *Wonder Women: Sex, Power, and the Quest for Perfection* (New York: Sarah Crichton Books, 2013).

2   A. Konar, N. Shah, R. Singh, N. Saxena, S. C. Kaul, R. Wadhwa, and M. K. Thakur. "Protective role of ashwagandha leaf extract and its component withanone on scopolamine-induced changes in the brain and brain-derived cells." *PLoS ONE* 6, no. 11 (2011): e27265. http://doi.org/10.1371/journal .pone.0027265.

3   N. Singh, M. Bhalla, P. de Jager, and M. Gilca. "An overview on ashwagandha: a Rasayana (rejuvenator) of Ayurveda." *African Journal of Traditional, Complementary, and Alternative Medicines* 8, no. 5 (Suppl) (2011): 208–13. http://doi.org/10.4314/ajtcam.v8i5S.9.

4   E. M. Olsson, B. von Scheele, and A. G. Panossian. "A randomised, double-blind, placebo-controlled, parallel-group study of the standardised extract SHR-5 of the roots of *Rhodiola rosea* in the treatment of subjects with stress-related fatigue." *Planta Medica* 75, no. 2 (2009): 105–12.

5   P. Rossi, D. Buonocore, E. Altobelli, F. Brandalise, V. Cesaroni, D. Iozzi, E. Savino, and F. Marzatico. "Improving training condition assessment in endurance cyclists: effects of *Ganoderma lucidum* and *Ophiocordyceps sinensis* dietary supplementation." *Evidence-based Complementary and Alternative Medicine* 2014 (2014): 979613.

6   H. J. Kang, H. W. Baik, S. J. Kim, S. G. Lee, H. Y. Ahn, J. S. Park, S. J. Park, E. J. Jang, S. W. Park, J. Y. Choi, J. H. Sung, and S. M. Lee. "*Cordyceps militaris* enhances cell-mediated immunity in healthy Korean men." *Journal of Medicinal Food* 18, no. 10 (2015): 1164–72.

7   D. Armanini, C. Fiore, M. J. Mattarello, J. Bielenberg, and M. Palermo. "History of the endocrine effects of licorice." *Experimental and Clinical Endocrinology and Diabetes* 110, no. 6 (2002): 257–61.

8   P. Patak, H. S. Willenberg, and S. R. Bornstein. "Vitamin C is an important cofactor for both adrenal cortex and adrenal medulla." *Endocrine Research* 30, no. 4 (2004): 871–75.

CHAPTER 4: THE FEMME FATALE

1   Gloria Steinem. *Revolution from Within: A Book of Self-Esteem* (New York: Little, Brown, 1992).

CHAPTER 5: THE ETHEREAL

1   F. Bäckhed, H. Ding, T. Wang, L. V. Hooper, G. Y. Koh, A. Nagy, C. F. Semenkovich, and J. I. Gordon. "The gut microbiota as an environmental factor that regulates fat storage." *Proceedings of the National Academy of Sciences of the United States of America* 101, no. 44 (2004): 15718–23.

2   P. J. Turnbaugh, R. E. Ley, M. A. Mahowald, V. Magrini, E. R. Mardis, and J. I. Gordon. "An obesity-associated gut microbiome with increased capacity for energy harvest." *Nature* 444 (2006): 1027–31.

CHAPTER 6: FOOD FUNDAMENTALS

1   A. Chaix, A. Zarrinpar, P. Miu, and S. Panda. "Time-restricted feeding is a preventative and therapeutic intervention against diverse nutritional challenges." *Cell Metabolism* 20, no. 6 (2014): 991–1005.

2   D. S. Ludwig, J. A. Majzoub, A. Al-Zahrani, G. E. Dallal, I. Blanco, and S. B. Roberts. "High glycemic index foods, overeating, and obesity." *Pediatrics* 103 (1999): E26.

CHAPTER 7: EAT YOUR VEGETABLES

1   M. Rizwan, I. Rodriguez-Blanco, A. Harbottle, M. A. Birch-Machin, R. E. Watson, and L. E. Rhodes. "Tomato paste rich in lycopene protects against cutaneous photodamage in humans in vivo: a randomized controlled trial." *British Journal of Dermatology* 164, no. 1 (2011): 154–62.

2   E. S. Mackinnon, A. V. Rao, and L. G. Rao. "Dietary restriction of lycopene for a period of one month resulted in significantly increased biomarkers of oxidative stress and bone resorption in postmenopausal women." *Journal of Nutrition, Health and Aging* 15, no. 2 (2011): 133–38.

3   D. J. Lamport, C. L. Lawton, N. Merat, H. Jamson, K. Myrissa, D. Hofman, H. K. Chadwick, F. Quadt, J. D. Wightman, and L. Dye. "Concord grape juice, cognitive function, and driving performance: a 12-wk, placebo-controlled, randomized crossover trial in mothers of preteen children." *American Journal of Clinical Nutrition* 103, no. 3 (2016): 775–83.

4   C. Stauth and G. D. Khalsa. *Meditation as Medicine* (New York: Simon and Schuster, 2001), 22.

CHAPTER 8: THE PROTEIN PARADOX

1   T. J. Key, M. Thorogood, P. N. Appleby, and M. L. Burr. "Dietary habits and mortality in 11,000 vegetarians and health conscious people: results of a 17 year follow up." *BMJ* 313, no. 7060 (September 28, 1996): 775–79. PubMed PMID: 8842068; PubMed Central PMCID: PMC2352199.

2   K. L. Resch. "[Dietary Intervention Randomized Controlled Trial (DIRECT) group: weight loss with a low-carbohydrate, Mediterranean, or low-fat diet]." *Forschende Komplementärmedizin* 15, no. 6 (2008): 351–52.

3   M. C. Morris, J. Brockman, J. A. Schneider, Y. Wang, D. A. Bennett, C. C. Tangney, and O. van de Rest. "Association of seafood consumption, brain mercury level, and APOE ε4 status with brain neuropathology in older adults." *Journal of the American Medical Association* 315, no. 5 (2016): 489–97.

4   S. H. Zeisel. "Nutritional importance of choline for brain development." *Journal of the American College of Nutrition* 23, no. 6 (Suppl) (2004): 621S–626S.

5   B. A. Griffin. "Eggs: good or bad?" *Proceedings of the Nutrition Society* 75, no. 3 (2016): 259–64.

6   D. Swiatecka, A. Narbad, K. P. Ridgway, and H. Kostyra. "The study on the impact of glycated pea proteins on human intestinal bacteria." *International Journal of Food Microbiology* 145, no. 1 (2011): 267–72.

CHAPTER 9: FAT FEARS AND FETISHES

1 D. Wang and E. S. Mitchell. "Cognition and synaptic-plasticity related changes in aged rats supplemented with 8- and 10-carbon medium chain triglycerides." *PLoS One* 11, no. 8 (2016): e0160159.

2 T. F. O'Callaghan, H. Faulkner, S. McAuliffe, M. G. O'Sullivan, D. Hennessy, P. Dillon, K. N. Kilcawley, C. Stanton, and R. P. Ross. "Quality characteristics, chemical composition, and sensory properties of butter from cows on pasture versus indoor feeding systems." *Journal of Dairy Science* 99, no. 12 (2016): 9441–60.

3 A. C. Watras, A. C. Buchholz, R. N. Close, Z. Zhang, and D. A. Schoeller. "The role of conjugated linoleic acid in reducing body fat and preventing holiday weight gain." *International Journal of Obesity* (London) 31, no. 3 (2007): 481–87.

CHAPTER 10: THE CARBOHYDRATE QUESTION

1 University of Chicago Celiac Disease Center. "A brief history of celiac disease." *Impact* 7, no. 3 (2007): 1. https://www.cureceliacdisease.org/wp-content/uploads/SU07CeliacCtr.News_.pdf (accessed June 20, 2017).

2 Samsel, A. and S. Seneff (2015). "Glyphosate, pathways to modern diseases III: Manganese, neurological diseases, and associated pathologies." Surg Neurol Int 6: 45.

3 Freire, R. H., L. R. Fernandes, R. B. Silva, B. S. Coelho, L. P. de Araujo, L. S. Ribeiro, J. M. Andrade, P. M. Lima, R. S. Araujo, S. H. Santos, C. C. Coimbra, V. N. Cardoso and J. I. Alvarez-Leite (2016). "Wheat gluten intake increases weight gain and adiposity associated with reduced thermogenesis and energy expenditure in an animal model of obesity." *Int J Obes* (Lond) 40(3): 479–486.

4 F. R. Soares, R. de Oliveira Matoso, L. G. Teixeira, Z. Menezes, S. S. Pereira, A. C. Alves, N. V. Batista, A. M. de Faria, D. C. Cara, A. V. Ferreira, and J. I. Alvarez-Leite. "Gluten-free diet reduces adiposity, inflammation and insulin resistance associated with the induction of PPAR-alpha and PPAR-gamma expression." *Journal of Nutritional Biochemistry* 24, no. 6 (2013): 1105–11.

5 Biesiekierski, J. R., & Iven, J. (2015). Non-coeliac gluten sensitivity: piecing the puzzle together. *United European Gastroenterology Journal*, 3(2), 160–165. http://doi.org/10.1177/2050640615578388

6 V. G. Zanwar, S. V. Pawar, P. A. Gambhire, S. S. Jain, R. G. Surude, V. B. Shah, Q. Q. Contractor, and P. M. Rathi. "Symptomatic improvement with gluten restriction in irritable bowel syndrome: a prospective, randomized, double blinded placebo controlled trial." *Intestinal Research* 14, no. 4 (2016): 343–50.

7 V. Bonciolini, B. Bianchi, E. Del Bianco, A. Verdelli, and M. Caproni. "Cutaneous manifestations of non-celiac gluten sensitivity: clinical histological and immunopathological features." *Nutrients* 7, no. 9 (2015): 7798–805.

8 R. L. Wu, M. I. Vazquez-Roque, P. Carlson, D. Burton, M. Grover, M. Camilleri, and J. R. Turner. "Gluten-induced symptoms in diarrhea-predominant irritable bowel syndrome are associated with increased myosin light chain kinase activity and claudin-15 expression." *Laboratory Investigation* 97, no. 1 (2017): 14–23.

9 G. Casella, R. Pozzi, M. Cicognetti, F. Bachetti, G. Torti, M. Cadei, V. Villanacci, V. Baldini, and G. Bassotti. "Mood disorders and non-celiac gluten sensitivity." *Minerva Gastroenterologica e Dietologica* 63, no. 1 (2017): 32–37.

10 S. Dos Santos and F. Lioté. "Osteoarticular manifestations of celiac disease and non-celiac gluten hypersensitivity." *Joint, Bone, Spine* 84, no. 3 (2017): 263–66.

11 L. Greco, M. Gobbetti, R. Auricchio, R. Di Mase, F. Landolfo, F. Paparo, R. Di Cagno, M. De Angelis, C. G. Rizzello, A. Cassone, G. Terrone, L. Timpone, M. D'Aniello, M. Maglio, R. Troncone, and S. Auricchio. "Safety for patients with celiac disease of baked goods made of wheat flour hydrolyzed during food processing." *Clinical Gastroenterology and Hepatology* 9, no. 1 (2011): 24–29.

CHAPTER 11: THE SEDUCTION OF SUGAR

1 J. Ma, N. M. McKeown, S. J. Hwang, U. Hoffmann, P. F. Jacques, and C. S. Fox. "Sugar-sweetened beverage consumption is associated with change of visceral adipose tissue over 6 years of follow-up." *Circulation* 133, no. 4 (2016): 370–77.

2 Suez, J., T. Korem, D. Zeevi, G. Zilberman-Schapira, C. A. Thaiss, O. Maza, D. Israeli, N. Zmora, S. Gilad, A. Weinberger, Y. Kuperman, A. Harmelin, I. Kolodkin-Gal, H. Shapiro, Z. Halpern, E. Segal and

E. Elinav (2014). "Artificial sweeteners induce glucose intolerance by altering the gut microbiota." *Nature* 514(7521): 181–186.

3   J. Hebebrand, O. Albayrak, R. Adan, J. Antel, C. Dieguez, J. de Jong, G. Leng, J. Menzies, J. G. Mercer, M. Murphy, G. van der Plasse, and S. L. Dickson. "'Eating addiction,' rather than 'food addiction,' better captures addictive-like eating behavior." *Neuroscience and Biobehavioral Reviews* 47 (2014): 295–306.

4   M. Lenoir, F. Serre, L. Cantin, and S. H. Ahmed. "Intense sweetness surpasses cocaine reward." *PLoS One* 2, no. 8 (2007): e698.

5   N. M. Avena, P. Rada, and B. G. Hoebel. "Evidence for sugar addiction: behavioral and neurochemical effects of intermittent, excessive sugar intake." *Neuroscience and Biobehavioral Reviews* 32, no. 1 (2008): 20–39. http://doi.org/10.1016/j.neubiorev.2007.04.019.

6   P. Johnson and P. Kenny. "Dopamine D2 receptors in addiction-like reward dysfunction and compulsive eating in obese rats." *Nature Neuroscience* 13, no. 5 (2010): 635–41.

7   J. W. Grimm, R. Weber, J. Barnes, J. Koerber, K. Dorsey, and E. Glueck. "Brief exposure to novel or enriched environments reduces sucrose cue-reactivity and consumption in rats after 1 or 30 days of forced abstinence from self-administration." PLoS One 8, no. 1 (2013): e54164.

8   L. Codipietro, M. Ceccarelli, and A. Ponzone. "Breastfeeding or oral sucrose solution in term neonates receiving heel lance: a randomized, controlled trial." *Pediatrics* 122, no. 3 (2008): e716–21.

9   L. Strathearn. "Maternal neglect: oxytocin, dopamine and the neurobiology of attachment." *Journal of Neuroendocrinology* 23, no. 11 (2011): 1054–65.

PART III: THE SIX RS TO HEAL YOUR MIND

1   A. E. Capello and C. R. Markus. "Differential influence of the 5-HTTLPR genotype, neuroticism and real-life acute stress exposure on appetite and energy intake." *Appetite* 77 (2014): 83–93.

2   A. D. Smith, A. Fildes, L. Cooke, M. Herle, N. Shakeshaft, R. Plomin, and C. Llewellyn. "Genetic and environmental influences on food preferences in adolescence." *American Journal of Clinical Nutrition* 104, no. 2 (2016): 446–53. http://doi.org/10.3945/ajcn.116.133983.

CHAPTER 15: RESTORE YOUR BRAIN

1   V. J. Felitti, R. F. Anda, D. Nordenberg, D. F. Williamson, A. M. Spitz, V. Edwards, M. P. Koss, and J. S. Marks. "Relationship of childhood abuse and household dysfunction to many of the leading causes of death in adults. The Adverse Childhood Experiences (ACE) Study." *American Journal of Preventive Medicine* 14, no. 4 (1998): 245–58.

2   A. Bosy-Westphal, S. Hinrichs, K. Jauch-Chara, B. Hitze, W. Later, B. Wilms, U. Settler, A. Peters, D. Kiosz, and M. J. Muller. "Influence of partial sleep deprivation on energy balance and insulin sensitivity in healthy women." *Obesity Facts* 1, no. 5 (2008): 266–73.

3   M. P. St-Onge, A. McReynolds, Z. B. Trivedi, A. L. Roberts, M. Sy, and J. Hirsch. "Sleep restriction leads to increased activation of brain regions sensitive to food stimuli." *American Journal of Clinical Nutrition* 95, no. 4 (2012): 818–24.

4   K. Spiegel, E. Tasali, P. Penev, and E. Van Cauter. "Brief communication: sleep curtailment in healthy young men is associated with decreased leptin levels, elevated ghrelin levels, and increased hunger and appetite." *Annals of Internal Medicine* 141, no. 11 (2004): 846–50.

5   J. M. Mullington, N. S. Simpson, H. K. Meier-Ewert, and M. Haack. "Sleep loss and inflammation." *Best Practice and Research. Clinical Endocrinology and Metabolism* 24, no. 5 (2010): 775–84. http://doi.org/10.1016/j.beem.2010.08.014.

6   R. Leproult, G. Copinschi, O. Buxton, and E. Van Cauter. "Sleep loss results in an elevation of cortisol levels the next evening." *Sleep* 20, no. 10 (1997): 865–70.

7   A. Mohan, R. Sharma, and R. L. Bijlani. "Effect of meditation on stress-induced changes in cognitive functions." *Journal of Alternative and Complementary Medicine* 17, no. 3 (2011): 207–12.

8   J. D. Creswell, M. R. Irwin, L. J. Burklund, M. D. Lieberman, J. M. Arevalo, J. Ma, . . .C. Breen, and S. W. Cole. "Mindfulness-Based Stress Reduction training reduces loneliness and pro-inflammatory gene expression in older adults: a small randomized controlled trial." *Brain, Behavior, and Immunity* 26, no. 7 (2012): 1095–101. http://doi.org/10.1016/j.bbi.2012.07.006.

9   B. K. Hölzel, J. Carmody, M. Vangel, C. Congleton, S. M. Yerramsetti, T. Gard, and S. W. Lazar. "Mindfulness practice leads to increases in regional brain gray matter density." *Psychiatry Research* 191, no. 1 (2011): 36–43. http://doi.org/10.1016/j.pscychresns.2010.08.006.

10 J. L. Kristeller and C. B. Hallett. "An exploratory study of a meditation-based intervention for binge eating disorder." *Journal of Health Psychology* 4, no. 3 (1999): 357–63.

CHAPTER 18: RELEASE YOUR EMOTIONS

1 Rogan, M. T., K. S. Leon, D. L. Perez and E. R. Kandel (2005). "Distinct Neural Signatures for Safety and Danger in the Amygdala and Striatum of the Mouse." *Neuron* 46(2): 309-320.
2 Howard Hughes Medical Institute. "Learning How Not to Be Afraid: Summary." October 8, 2008. http://www.hhmi.org/news/learning-how-not-be-afraid (accessed August 21, 2017).
3 D. Church, G. Yount, and A. J. Brooks. "The effect of emotional freedom techniques on stress biochemistry: a randomized controlled trial." *Journal of Nervous and Mental Disease* 200, no. 10 (2012): 891–96.
4 D. Church, G. Yount, K. Rachlin, L. Fox, and J. Nelms. "Epigenetic effects of PTSD remediation in veterans using clinical emotional freedom techniques: a randomized controlled pilot study." *American Journal of Health Promotion* 32, no. 1 (2018): 112–22.
5 M. A. Katzman, M. Vermani, P. L. Gerberg, R. P. Brown, C. Iorio, M. Davis, C. Cameron, . . .and D. Tsirgielis. "A multicomponent yoga-based, breath intervention program as an adjunctive treatment in patients suffering from generalized anxiety disorder with or without comorbidities." *International Journal of Yoga* 5, no. 1 (2012): 57–65.
6 H. Lavretsky, E. S. Epel, P. Siddarth, N. Nazarian, N. S. Cyr, D. S. Khalsa, J. Lin, E. Blackburn, and M. R. Irwin. "A pilot study of yogic meditation for family dementia caregivers with depressive symptoms: effects on mental health, cognition, and telomerase activity." *International Journal of Geriatric Psychiatry* 28, no. 1 (2013): 57–65. http://doi.org/10.1002/gps.3790.

CHAPTER 20: REVIVE YOUR SENSE OF SELF

1 S. W. Cole. "Social regulation of human gene expression." *Current Directions in Psychological Science* 18, no. 3 (2009): 132–37. http://doi.org/10.1111/j.1467-8721.2009.01623.x.
2 http://www.npr.org/sections/health-shots/2015/11/29/457255876/loneliness-may-warp-our-genes -and-our-immune-systems.
3 H. Woolhouse, A. Knowles, and N. Crafti. "Adding mindfulness to CBT programs for binge eating: a mixed-methods evaluation." *Eating Disorders* 20, no. 4 (2012): 321–39. doi: 10.1080/10640266 .2012.691791. PubMed PMID: 22703573.

INDEX

====

ABOUT THE AUTHOR

Dana James MS, CNS, CDN, received her masters of science in medical nutrition from Columbia University. She is a board-certified nutritionist, functional medicine practitioner. and cognitive behavioral therapist. She specializes in weight loss, woman's hormonal health, mood disorders, and destigmatizing shame from childhood experiences. She is a trusted nutrition and self-worth expert for media outlets like *The New York Times, Elle, Vogue, Harper's Bazaar,* and MindBodyGreen. She divides her time between New York City and Los Angeles.